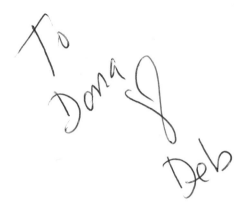

# Says Who?

"Rooted in the liberating Buddhist principle, "What we believe, we become," Ora's wise and timely book presents a clear and simple method—a series of seven insightful and revealing questions—to not only identify self-limiting thoughts but to mindfully challenge and transform them into insight, passion, and freedom—the requisites that help us achieve our goals while living in peace and dignity in the process."

—**Alan Clements**, author of *A Future To Believe In* and *The Voice of Hope: Conversations with Burma's Nobel Laureate, Aung San Suu Kyi.*

# Says Who?

*How One Simple
Question Can Change
the Way You
Think Forever*

## Ora Nadrich

New York

# Says Who?

## *How One Simple Question Can Change the Way You Think Forever*

© 2016 Ora Nadrich.

Published in New York, New York, by Morgan James Publishing. Morgan James and The Entrepreneurial Publisher are trademarks of Morgan James, LLC.
www.MorganJamesPublishing.com

The Morgan James Speakers Group can bring authors to your live event. For more information or to book an event visit The Morgan James Speakers Group at
www.TheMorganJamesSpeakersGroup.com.

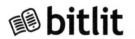

A **free** eBook edition is available
with the purchase of this print book.

CLEARLY PRINT YOUR NAME ABOVE IN UPPER CASE

**Instructions to claim your free eBook edition:**
1. Download the BitLit app for Android or iOS
2. Write your name in **UPPER CASE** on the line
3. Use the BitLit app to submit a photo
4. Download your eBook to any device

ISBN 978-1-63047-627-4  paperback
Library of Congress Control Number:
2015906044

**Cover Photograph by**
Denise Malone

**Cover Design by:**
Rachel Lopez
www.r2cdesign.com

**Interior Design by:**
Bonnie Bushman
The Whole Caboodle Graphic Design

In an effort to support local communities and raise awareness and funds, Morgan James Publishing donates a percentage of all book sales for the life of each book to Habitat for Humanity Peninsula and Greater Williamsburg.

Get involved today, visit
www.MorganJamesBuilds.com

**Habitat**
**for Humanity®**
Peninsula and
Greater Williamsburg
Building Partner

# Table of Contents

# Acknowledgements

I wish to thank the following very special people in my life who have been an important part of my journey. My loving and encouraging husband, Jeff, who is the rock of our family, and my two amazing sons, Jake and Benjamin, who are a blessing to me. Your understanding of my process in doing the work that moves my soul means so much to me. I love you very much. My beloved mother, Dora, who has always valued helping people, which I feel I inherited. You are such an incredible inspiration to me. My trailblazer sister, Nesa, who has always championed me. My sister, Esty, whose profound story set me on a life changing path to understand our thoughts better, which inspired the writing of this book. My beautiful niece, Sarah, who makes me feel so appreciated. Kathleen Felesina, who was there from the very beginning when I had the idea to write *Says Who?* and was such a great editor. Harriet Friedman, who has helped me "individuate" and come to know myself better than I could have ever imagined. Dr. Ronald Alexander, who has mentored me so magnificently on the Mindfulness Meditation path. Alan Clements, who encouraged me to keep the integrity of my book as I released it out into the world. Marianne Williamson, who believed in me and my book. My wonderful girlfriends who have been there for me with their love and valued friendships. And finally, in memoriam, David Z. Goodman, who always told me I was a writer, and my father, Simon, and brother, Daniel, both wise and deeply spiritual, and whose spirits I feel guide me, strengthening my belief in what isn't always seen, but what my heart tells me is true and most real.

# Introduction

*Rule your mind or it will rule you.*
**—Horace**

## A Search for Answers

I had one of those stable, wonderful childhoods that people yearn for. The youngest of four children, I have vivid memories of endless laughter in our home, lively family dinners, and how much I loved playing with my sisters and brother. I skipped and did cartwheels almost as much as I walked, which clearly indicates a happy little girl. In fact, whenever I run into one of my childhood friends nowadays, they'll often say, "I always wished I was in your family. Some of my best memories as a child are from your house! There was so much warmth and closeness."

And it was true. I idolized my two beautiful sisters, as did my friends, and my brother was very special to me. My father was hard working, having come to America from Eastern Europe as a gourmet pastry chef, and my mother was truly perfect in my eyes. I always felt loved, never overshadowed by my homecoming queen sister or dean's list brother. Ever the actress in my family, I would spend hours dancing around the house and making up plays. When I announced at age twelve that I was going to be a professional actress when I grew up, I got total support and encouragement, especially from my mother who had the talent to become an opera singer, but chose family over career. I had the confidence and belief in myself that my supportive home life provided. I felt there was nothing I couldn't do.

At age fourteen, however, those feelings utterly vanished. I had no idea that those halcyon days of my childhood were simply that—the calm before the storm, or, in my family's case, a devastating tsunami. Shortly after my fourteenth birthday, my sister had a sudden, devastating nervous breakdown.

## Rough Seas

Three years older than me, my sister had always been stunningly beautiful, with a magnetic personality to match. Her charisma and independent spirit drew everyone to her and created excitement wherever she went— she was popular and fearless and I wanted to be just like her.

Then, just like that, the sister I knew and looked up to one day was suddenly gone the next, replaced by a manic, delusional, erratic being who ranted about voices in her head and completely turned life as I knew it upside down. Her life would never be the same and neither would mine. I went from a world where everything had a semblance of order to complete chaos. It was shocking.

In those first few months, as she moved from hospital to psych ward to halfway house to home again, I was pretty much shell-shocked, as were my parents, who were also reeling and too overwhelmed to actually sit me down and explain things. I heard the terms "schizophrenia" and "manic depressive" almost in passing, not really knowing what they meant. Yet I did understand that things were never going to be the same again, for my sister or any of us. This wasn't just a temporary break with reality for her but a lifelong condition—a realization even more devastating than her initial breakdown. It was almost like a death.

Salvation and escape came through my imaginary world where I felt most comfortable—acting. It was a wonderful place to go; getting lost in another character gave me respite from the all too real trauma and devastation of my sister's illness and the upheaval it caused in my family. This was the world for me, my calling.

So after high school, while I spent a couple of years in college taking writing and psychology courses, I also spent as much time in acting classes and making the rounds of auditions. I was always comfortable expressing myself and emoting and this seemed the perfect outlet for me. I even mentally prepared myself for the possibility of years of obscurity as an actress waiting for her break. That's why it was such a pleasant and gratifying surprise when things started happening for me fairly quickly. My appearance in a USC student film led to my landing an agent and, before I knew it, my first role in a film: *Altered States*, with William Hurt. My part was small, but it soon led to other things: TV roles and commercial work. I was a working actress! Then the film came out and was a success. Suddenly I was part of the Hollywood social scene, meeting and auditioning with some of the best actors of the day. I started reading for some pretty big parts. I was really on my way.

Then the letters started coming.

I had been so focused on my acting classes and auditions that I hadn't really thought about the prospect of notoriety or fan mail, but when it started coming shortly after *Altered States* came out, instead of flattering me, the attention had the opposite effect. It gave me anxiety.

Acting had gone from being a salvation to a fear. Although the anxious feelings would ebb and flow, they never really went away. I went from confident and comfortable in my own skin to second-guessing myself and being uncertain. Suddenly I didn't feel secure enough to deal with the outside forces and the prospect of constant exposure of being an actress.

Part of it had to do with my sister. I had obviously never resolved the fears and shock from her breakdown, not to mention the guilt. I was plagued by doubts and questions like, *Why is my life (and mind) working and hers isn't? Am I going to become like her one day?* My survival mechanism had pushed down and suppressed those feelings up until then, but the sudden attention my blossoming acting career brought seemed to cause those thoughts to bubble up and it was taking its toll. I had taken enough psychology classes and read enough self-help books to know that I needed help.

## Journey of Self Discovery

Thus began my lifelong journey to understand the mind better. I wanted to know:

*Why am I thinking these thoughts?*
*Why am I feeling these feelings?*
*What are these anxious thoughts about?*
*What is causing my increasing panic, as if I was standing at the edge of a cliff looking down, and could easily fall off?*
*Why do I feel so out of control?*
*Can I do anything about it?*

These questions plagued me constantly. Not only that, but I was also beginning to feel like I was walking a few feet off the ground, and nothing was anchoring me to the earth. I felt more and more powerless—terrified that this feeling of being out of control meant that I was one step away from losing my grip on reality, like my sister, and having a nervous breakdown, never to recover.

Even though I had tried so hard to learn how to cope with my sister's illness, I realized I hadn't truly been aware of how much her breakdown had affected me profoundly, and that I too suffered a serious trauma of my own. Now that trauma was starting to take control over my life, interrupting my deepest passion and focus—acting. I was definitely grappling with my own mental and emotional well being, and if I didn't get professional help to understand what was happening to me, I knew my fate could possibly end up being as unfortunate as hers.

Thankfully, because of the months of family therapy we'd participated in after my sister's breakdown and the psych classes I took in college, I had a bit of knowledge at least about where to begin. My first step in what was to become an all encompassing psycho-spiritual journey for the next fifteen years was to go to a cognitive therapist.

**Cognitive behavioral therapy (CBT)** is a form of psychotherapy in which the therapist and the client work together as a team to identify, solve, and overcome their problems by understanding their thinking, behavior, and emotional responses. It's designed to help you comprehend your thoughts better so that you can get to the root of what causes your fears and anxieties, particularly through understanding where these thoughts come from in the first place.

I found an excellent CBT therapist, who, through asking me a series of questions, would help me trace the origins of where each of my anxiety-ridden, fear-based thoughts began. So if I said something like, "I'm feeling anxious and the world seems frightening to me," he would then ask, "What specifically is making you feel anxious?" and "What in particular about the world frightens you?"

In the beginning I would tell him more about what I was feeling rather than the specific thoughts I was having around my feelings because at the time I was interpreting everything emotionally through a prism of anxiety. That is, I was aware of my *feelings*, but I didn't yet know that certain *thoughts* were the reason I was feeling the way I was, particularly the underlying belief that I could have a nervous breakdown like my sister. Though this thought was at the bottom of everything I was experiencing, I hadn't connected it directly yet as the reason for my fear and anxiety. I was too busy *reacting* to my thoughts, not trying to understand them. My mind was defaulting to what I eventually learned were *automatic thoughts*—like the thoughts of guilt and panic that would pop up sometimes as a result of how I felt about my sister's crisis—and I was simply reacting to them, operating directly on impulse.

However, simply talking about my fears with him didn't alleviate all of the anxiety I was still experiencing. It was helpful to talk to a therapist about what was bothering me, and introduced the ability to question my thoughts, which I found very interesting and planted a seed in me about the importance of understanding how we think, but I knew I had to go further and deeper into myself to know my entire being, which is what I was really longing for.

It was then that I embarked on what became a two-decade quest for knowledge and understanding of how our thoughts work and how to manage them. During those years I went on to study many more psychological and spiritual modalities and techniques. I also began practicing Transcendental Meditation and Hatha Yoga, which opened up a deep interest for me in Buddhism.

All of the techniques I learned were eye opening and very illuminating. I was definitely on a quest for self-exploration, inner peace and knowledge, and I wanted to know everything I could about who I am and what my purpose is. Something deep within me kept pushing me forward on this quest like it was my destiny and I shouldn't be afraid.

## An Awakening

Even as I continued on my spiritual quest, though, I still felt an underlying feeling of anxiety from time to time. This signaled to me that, even with all of the incredible things I was discovering on my journey of self-realization, I knew I needed something even deeper and more psychologically oriented to get to the bottom of what was causing my anxiety and fear. I decided to go into Jungian analysis.

Jungian analysis was an extraordinary revelation. Discovering the brilliant wisdom of Carl Jung, the founder of analytical psychology, was exactly what I needed. From the minute I walked into my therapist's office, I knew that I was in the right place. I'd read several Jungian psychology books before, which resonated with me immediately, so I intuitively knew that whatever I was experiencing in my mind, as frightening as it was, Jung's teachings could help me understand it better. But never did I imagine that I would be embarking on a journey that would literally turn my psyche inside out, allowing me to come face to face with all of my fears and anxiety, and that by analyzing my dreams as well, which is an integral part of Jungian therapy, I would come to know myself better than I would ever have imagined was possible.

I believe in divine providence, and that when you are ready and truly ask for something you need so desperately, you will find it. For me it was Jungian analysis. I needed a type of psychology that could help me understand who I am fully, and for me that meant knowing myself separate from anyone else, especially a sister who had a promising life tragically derailed by mental illness. I wanted to know who I am as a unique individual (which each of us are) separate from her; to discover how, even though she and I were from the same biological family and share genes, I have a particular destiny to fulfill, and must live my life as it was meant solely for me. But in order for me to realize that, I first had to untangle my enmeshment with my sister and her illness, and find my healthy, authentic self, which was getting buried under the darkness of her misfortune.

Jung called identifying your true, inner self, distinct from others the **Individuation Process**. It's living all parts of who you are, and becoming awake to your true nature, which is beyond the limitations and fears we place on ourselves. I felt that underneath my fear was my true self wanting to be free of what was having power over me, which was my sister's illness, and this was the problem I was having: seeing myself "distinct," or separate from her. When I went into Jungian analysis, I thought that I "could" become like my sister, as if her mental illness was contagious, or that I, like her, was pre-disposed to getting a mental illness. These were some of the many thoughts I had at the time, and they were supported by my fear of that very dark incident. That darkness was taking me over, overshadowing other things in my life that were good, positive, and life affirming. I also carried around for many years "survivors guilt"—that it was my job to help her, and to somehow fix this terrible mistake that happened to her, as if it was my responsibility to reverse her fate. It was an incredible burden I had placed on myself, and it was those kinds of thoughts that kept me feeling so out of control, becoming the major cause of my anxiety.

Outwardly it seemed like I was coping just fine, but the combination of the fear I had over my sister's breakdown, coupled with more fear that it could happen to me, along with the added pressure to "fix it," created a thinking pattern that kept me in a constant state of worry and a feeling of anxiousness. My life had become inexorably linked with hers, and even though I seemed to be functioning just fine and probably no one knew that I was suffering inside, this was the reality I was living with. Jungian analysis helped me understand all of this. It shined a light on the idea of how you can remain stuck in your life when you don't know yourself as fully separate from others.

By continuing to probe further into my mind and examine my thoughts, I finally came to understand that in order for me to be able to live the life I was meant to, I must change the way I think and become individuated—in other words, discover my true, authentic self, separate from others' problems or misfortunes. I suddenly felt determined to be free and unburdened by things that didn't belong to me, to no longer carry other people's pain or suffering on my back, which can become the "baggage" we take on as our own. My sister had become that painful "baggage" I was carrying around. No one put her terrible misfortune on me other than myself, and it was time for me to separate myself from it, and release her to her own fate, as tragic as it was, which had nothing to do with me. Yes, I will forever mourn the loss of the beautiful, loving sister with the great spirited laugh that made everyone feel more alive when they were near her when she was well, but I can now hold the precious memory of who she once was in a special place in my heart, and no longer live in the past of what was, or could have been, or supposed to be. This was the "new thinking" I was allowing for in my mind. The realization that I could change old thoughts mired in fear and anxiety into healthy ones that are positive, and not fear-based, was liberating and life changing for me. And I understood that the most effective way to do that was to question my thoughts.

## Questioning Our Thoughts

It wasn't until after many years of my psycho-spiritual exploring that I came to understand and believe that by **questioning our thoughts**, we *can* know them better, and by knowing them better, we can determine what purpose they serve for us, whether negative or positive, and that we are in complete control of deciding what thoughts we can accept or release, which ultimately affects our well-being. Keeping negative thoughts in our mind allows them to fester, and have a greater hold on us, which then increases whatever anxiety or fear is already there, and when we're functioning out of anxiety and fear, we are that much more susceptible to believing our negative thoughts, even if they aren't true. This creates a vicious cycle that can become extremely difficult to break, which is exactly what had happened to me. I believed my fear based thoughts because I didn't know that I could question them, but when I finally did because I was sick and tired of being at the affect of them, I found out they weren't real, and it was then that I realized with absolute certainty that I had the power to remove them from my mind.

This was my "gestalt," which is a psychological term meaning you take personal responsibility for what you discover and realize about yourself, and make serious adjustments because of it. It's the great epiphany, or the "aha" moment, that changes the way you think about something entirely.

Before then I accepted all my thoughts as "real," and never questioned them. The thought that "I could have a breakdown like my sister," without questioning it with something as logical as "Why do I think that?" or, "Did someone tell me I was going to have a breakdown like my sister?" or, "Do I have to have a breakdown like my sister?" was not a part of my thinking process, and never did I once think to even challenge my fearful thoughts so they remained in my mind, undermining my well-being and distorting my perception of myself. But by questioning them, I could challenge those very perceptions and the thoughts themselves. I didn't just accept them anymore—I confronted them, questioned their origins to determine if they were "real" or simply automatic negative thoughts that served no useful purpose whatsoever. This practice is what finally helped shift my mind from reverting back to those futile, fear-based thoughts, and kept me on a positive, healthy thinking track with consistency.

## Knowing Our Thoughts

Whether or not our perceptions are accurate or correct can only be determined by our questioning of them so that we can get to what is real or based in reality. Cognition is "the process or act of knowing." We come to "know" things by how we "perceive" them. You can correct distorted thinking by taking a closer look at how faulty or unrealistic you're thinking is—which in my case was the nagging thought that I could have a nervous breakdown like my sister—by simply asking questions designed to get at the root of your process of thinking. There was nothing substantive or concrete to back that thought up other than my mind functioning out of *fear* and *emotion* because of what had happened to her, so whatever thoughts I had while I was in that constant state of fear would invariably be distorted. If I could back the thought that I could become mentally ill like my sister with a thought like "statistics and data prove that siblings have the exact same mental health outcome as each other," then I could justify my fear and anxiety, but that was clearly not the case. It was by questioning and challenging my thoughts that I came to know them better, and was able to distinguish between which were real, and which were not.

## Becoming a Life Coach

Understanding better how we think remained my passion as I continued further on my journey. I stopped acting, eventually got married and had children, and continued studying and learning more about the workings of the mind. Knowing who we are in this lifetime seemed like the most valuable and important thing we can do, and to "individuate" or become fully awake to ourselves is truly possible for everyone, if they desire it. I wanted to help others awaken to themselves too, like I had. It was so liberating and life changing for me, but I knew that not everyone has the time or means to do it through therapy like I did.

I always loved helping people when they were having a hard time or going through difficulties, even in my days as an actress, and aside from them telling me that I always made them feel better and helped them get through whatever they were dealing with, I knew it was my ability to ask them specific, almost tailor-made questions about what they "thought" about their situation that was the most effective and useful to them. Just talking about your problems, and doing nothing about them, is ultimately useless. It won't help you during those times when your thoughts can make you feel like you're stuck on a hamster wheel, spinning negativity with no real way to make that thinking process stop or reverse it. But, if you can stop your negative thinking process, then you can genuinely change the pattern of your unhappiness that is directly linked to the thoughts you have. It's all about "re-thinking," and I yearned to have people know how easy it really is to do.

So I decided to take it from being the "friend in need" to becoming a certified Life Coach, where I could professionally help people and teach them how to question their own thoughts like I had learned to do. Questioning and knowing how our thoughts work became the cornerstone of my Life Coaching, and the basis of the unique method I've developed that I use with great effect with both my private clients as well as in the various workshops and women's groups I facilitate. My method, which begins and revolves around a simple question—"Says Who?" –comes from distilling nearly twenty years of delving into the mind and exploring various methods and modalities for cognitive and spiritual clarity into a very simple, effective and practical process, which I will explain in the following chapters that I've been using on my clients ever since.

Essentially, with this method, my clients saw, in a relatively short time, that I was able to take them from staying stuck in how they "think" about their problems, to empowering them to be able to question their thoughts—to know which ones are positive and real, and which ones are negative and not real, and that all of their thoughts should serve their well being. Soon they were having their own "aha" moments, which led to profound shifts in their consciousness and the way they handled the inevitable obstacles in their lives. Most satisfying of all was how this method could work on anyone—it applies to young and old, male and female, with problems big and small, and I am thrilled to share with you in this book this very effective technique I've created.

The *Says Who?* method is a wonderful "go to" set of specific questions that you can ask yourself anytime, anywhere. I encourage you to learn it by heart and use it in whatever situation you find yourself when you feel fear, doubt, or diminished in any way. Those states of mind are often not "real," and can be changed instantly with these simple set of questions designed to challenge and reconstruct your thinking. With time and practice, this method will become second nature for you, allowing you to nip a negative or fear-based thought in the bud. This new way of thinking, which I believe is the "correct" way to think, will become your natural thought process, and you will quickly detect when your thinking is distorted and be able to change it.

As you will see in the following chapters, to begin the process I have consolidated the questions into seven of what I feel are the most user-friendly and effective. The very first question, "Says who?" will stop your negative thought in its tracks whenever it pops up in your head, and expose it for exactly what it is—disruptive and potentially damaging to your well-being, and the following six questions will examine them even further and help resolve them.

Remember, your thoughts belong to no one, but you. Make them what you want them to be. You are the creator and master of your internal dialogue, which creates your reality.

## PART I

# Know Your
# Thoughts

*What we think, we become.*
**—Buddha**

*A man who does not think for himself does not think at all.*
**—Oscar Wilde**

# Chapter 1

# How Well Do You
# Know Your Thoughts?

*The world we have created is a product of our thinking.*
*It cannot be changed without changing our thinking.*
**—Albert Einstein**

A recent statistic claims we can think up to 70,000 thoughts per day. That's quite a lot of thoughts!

But how well do we know our thoughts? You may think, "Of course I know my thoughts! I'm the one having them!" But just being aware that you're having thoughts is not the same as *knowing* them— that is, their origin, how they affect you, whether they are reasonable and realistic, or even whether you can have power over them.

Have you ever considered questioning your thoughts, or do you just accept whatever comes into your head as normal thinking? Since we have so many thousands of thoughts per day, many of which are bound to be negative, do you know how you would even begin to question them or know which ones to challenge (or whether to challenge them)?

Most of us probably don't think about questioning our thoughts. But, if even half of our thoughts we think each day are negative, it's easy to see how letting those thoughts exist unchecked and unquestioned can make staying positive, productive and goal-oriented difficult.

The reason: a particular thought can pop up, and it gets our attention more than the others, especially if it's negative. That's usually because we have some kind of energy or an emotion around it, and it just doesn't seem to go away. Even if it recedes somewhere to the back of our mind, it will usually pop up again, sometimes when we least expect it, especially in times of stress, agitation or flux.

A thought that doesn't go away is a thought that's trying to tell you something more than just what's on the surface. And if you don't pay attention to it, it's probably going to stick around and make sure that you do. That isn't a problem if it's a productive thought like reminding you to pay a bill, or call a parent you haven't spoken to recently, for instance, but if it's a recurring thought that's negative or causing anxiety for no apparent reason, that can be an issue.

So how can we know what a thought is trying to tell us if we don't question it? The answer is, we can't. The only way we can know what a thought is trying to convey is by questioning it, and that means finding out where it came from, what it's doing there, and what purpose it serves for your well being. A positive thought is useful and productive, and makes you feel good about yourself. Recurring negative thoughts do nothing but make you feel bad and diminished in some way, and most often hold no purpose in serving your well-being. Yet many people will accept those kinds of thoughts as real and hold on to them, whether they are based in reality or not.

For instance, people suffering from anorexia steadfastly hold onto the thought that they are fat, even when they can see their skeletal frames in the mirror. While that is an extreme case, it is an example of how strong and pervasive a negative thought can take root in our minds, convincing us that they're real, even if the mirror says otherwise.

So how do you question a thought that makes you feel bad, and find out whether it's based on what is real, or is instead an inaccurate or distorted perception because of an experience you've had in the past that was negative, and influenced your thinking as a result?

## The Origins of "Says Who?"

From the very beginning of my practice I tried various ways and methods with my clients to encourage them to question and challenge their thoughts as the way to push through and address what was holding them back. I tried various types of questions and modes of inquiry to get them to become aware of how their thoughts worked and where they originated as a way to come up with a solution to whatever was bothering them. While this process was effective and my clients made progress, I still had a lingering feeling that there was a more streamlined, effective way to get to the root of our thoughts. Then, one day, I had my own breakthrough.

Not too long after I started coaching I began to notice a pattern with my clients. The beliefs they held about themselves that invariably caused them the most grief were often those that weren't based on their own original thoughts; that is, they were opinions of others they had listened to and accepted as their own.

So when my clients would say things like, "I'm afraid I'm going to fail," or "I'm not successful at relationships," or "I'm never going to realize my dreams," my own exploration into overcoming my fear-based thoughts, helped me realize that these negative thoughts they held about themselves that would invariably pop up, whenever they felt anxiety or insecurity or ran into some sort of obstacle in their lives, were often not even their own. These thoughts would then become a part of their belief system. They never challenged or questioned them, never thought, *Do I have to think that about myself?* They just accepted it as true. And then it occurred to me to ask, why wouldn't you want to challenge or question a belief about yourself that's causing unhappiness and making you feel bad about yourself/insecure/less than? Why wouldn't you want to find out the source of why you hold that negative belief about yourself?

One day I was counseling a new client who was dealing with those types of negative, nagging thoughts; those second-guessing, self-sabotaging thoughts, such as the belief that any risk or chance she took in her career was going to mean she was going to fail and lose everything. It was an extreme view that had little evidence to support it, especially since she was a very smart, talented, capable woman, yet those thoughts were holding her back from taking the positive steps she needed to reach her goals professionally. She was stuck.

"I know I'm going to end up in the poorhouse!" she kept saying, as if it was going to happen any minute. I was used to extreme or exaggerated feelings and concerns like these from my clients, and how they would let negativity fester in their minds without ever even considering challenging it to find out if it was based in fact, or simply fear. But what struck me as curious about this particular client was that, with her new business starting off so well, she clearly was on an upwardly mobile trajectory. So why would this negative thought, which was in direct opposition to the positive "reality" she was experiencing, have this kind of power over her? It was as if there were two minds working concurrently, yet in direct opposition with one another—a phenomenon I often saw with clients who were doing well. There was a part of their thinking that wasn't supporting their forward progress, and was actually trying to undermine or sabotage their positive efforts.

As she continued to profess with certainty her negative belief that she was destined to end up penniless—despite all evidence to the contrary—I came to the conclusion, with equal certainty, that I was not going to let her accept her negative belief as true for her, and I wanted her to know that, in no uncertain terms. It was crystal clear to me that I had to do something to challenge her thoughts to get her to change her thinking, and not accept that negative belief about herself.

"Says who?" I asked her, suddenly. The question literally popped out of my mouth before I could even think. Yet, in a way, it was exactly the type of question I had long wanted to ask my clients when they would get stuck believing their negative thoughts (that often didn't originate with them) that were holding them back. Those negative thoughts were frequently the result of something someone else, like a critical parent, insensitive teacher, or angry partner, said to them at some point in their life, and they believed it without ever thinking to question or challenge it.

My client looked at me curiously, like she wasn't quite sure what I was asking her. I took it further. "*Who* said that you're not going to be successful and end up in the poorhouse? Have you heard someone say this before?"

She thought about it long and hard. I kept going. I knew I was onto something.

"Did you ever consider that the negative, defeating thoughts you're experiencing now might not have originated with you, and that it was someone else's thoughts or opinions?"

She looked at me like I had just turned a light on in her head.

"Maybe," I said, "you've been walking around with this criticism and judgment of yourself for years and it's not even your own?"

I saw my challenge percolate in her mind, followed by a gradual dawning of awareness. It was her "aha moment," happening right in front of me.

"You know," she said in a stunned voice, "my father always used to say 'we're going to end up in the poorhouse' when we were kids. I never made the connection until now!"

"So those were his thoughts then, right?" I asked her.

"Yes, they were his, and it always bothered me when he would say it. It would actually scare me as a little kid. I thought we were going to end up on the street without a home."

"Did that ever happen?" I asked.

She shook her head and softly said, "No."

"Can you see," I explained, "how you took on your father's fearful thinking and made it your own, which became a belief?"

"Yes, but I don't want to think that way!" She declared emphatically.

"That's good," I told her. "Because you don't have to. Replace your father's negative thoughts with your own positive thoughts about yourself."

She laughed, and said, "You make it sound so easy."

"It is," I said. "Hard to believe, but it's true."

Within a fairly short time my client found the confidence to work toward her goal of launching her new business, which took off and is doing well. Even though negative and defeating thoughts still pop up for her from time to time—it's unrealistic to think you can banish negativity forever—she now reports that she is much better equipped to identify and deal with them. The set of questions I designed for her during those sessions, which became the basis of my method, allowed her to see how certain thoughts were not her own original thoughts and were not based in fact. By questioning and challenging her thoughts, she was able to learn how to not allow negative thoughts or beliefs to overtake her and derail her from her goals.

This method, which I refined and soon began to use with my other clients with great success, created for me my own "aha moment" as well. It was amazing how one simple question, followed by a series of follow-up questions, was able to create a shift in thinking rather quickly; how the very exercise of challenging a negative thought created a transformation that enabled my clients to have more control over their thoughts. Once they knew they were in control of changing their negative thoughts, they were eager to keep doing it because the results made them feel more confident, positive and in charge of their lives. It was exciting and liberating.

From there I was able to develop a very simple yet effective method that, by asking themselves a proscribed set of questions whenever a negative thought or series of thoughts popped up, would allow my clients to attack the problem proactively and keep it from derailing them from their goal, whether it be losing weight, changing careers, becoming a better parent or spouse, dealing with loss or any of the myriad issues that plague us and cause negativity to rear its ugly head.

We've come to know that our thoughts create our beliefs, which then affects our behavior. When my clients would tell me that when they changed their negative thoughts to ones that were more positive and productive, they would feel happier and more motivated, I wasn't surprised. This new-found shift for them in their thinking would allow them to build a more constructive and affirmative path toward their goals, without the fear of uncontrollable negative thoughts lurking in the background (such as those I used to have about my sister's illness), threatening to bring them down.

I found that the first question I had my clients ask themselves after *Says Who?*—"Have I heard someone say this before?"—helped establish where the thoughts came from, which then helped determine whether the thoughts were original, or just the opinions and beliefs of others that they took on as their own. And even if it was determined that the negative thought was their own, the method was still very effective at tracking the source of their negativity. By taking responsibility for it, they could overcome it.

To know that we are in control of who we are and everything we think, and can change our thinking to be exactly what we want it to be, is a very compelling and empowering concept. However, it's not as easy as snapping your fingers to change years of familiar habits and patterns of thought. While the *Says Who?* method provides the catalyst for examining our thoughts, I've found that, in order for the method to be successful, it not only must become a new "healthy" habit, but that it is imperative to genuinely want to know more about how our thoughts originate and how they work, as well as the different types of thoughts—positive and negative—we have. It is the willingness to explore what I like to call the "truth of our thoughts" (what our thoughts really want us to know) that is necessary and essential for the *Says Who?* method to work effectively.

I've culled the relevant and most important information concerning how our thoughts work, and distilled it in the following chapters in Part One, which provides a thorough examination of the thought process. This section of the book is labeled "Know Your Thoughts" to drive home the point that unless we question our thoughts, especially the ones that are negative, fear-based or diminishing of who we are, we cannot know our thoughts completely, which means that we are not in control of them—they are in control of us. If you want to be in the driver's seat of your life, and manifest your own "original" reality, which means your truth and vision of the life you want to live, you must know your thoughts, and that means all of them—positive *and* negative. By doing this, you can remove the negative thoughts that are impeding you from creating the positive life you desire.

Part Two, "Acknowledge Your Thoughts" takes you through the process of how to become an observer and not a reactor to your thoughts, so you can better work the method in a more effective fashion. Part Three, "Transform Your Thoughts", deals with how to incorporate the method into your life and make it more of a daily practice in order to reshape your thinking to be in alignment with your desires. Remember, you are the gatekeeper of your mind, and can decide what you want to let in—and what you don't.

## Chapter 2

# How Our Thoughts
# Influence Our Lives

*The more man meditates upon good thoughts,
the better will be his world and the world at large.*
**—Confucius**

I
t goes without saying that our thoughts influence every single
thing in our lives. They determine what we feel about ourselves,
others, and the world, and what we express about our beliefs,
opinions, values and judgments. Because our thoughts are formed by
how we perceive things, depending on our experiences—positive or
negative—our ideas and attitudes about everything are based on how
we are not only *affected* by those experiences, but by how we *interpret*
those experiences.

An example of this would be when you were young and someone—a
teacher, sibling, friend or even complete stranger—told you or gave

you the impression that you weren't "good enough" at something, be it singing, dancing, school, basketball, or whatever. Until that person said that to you, or made you feel that way, you might not have thought that about yourself, but now that someone else's thought has made its way into your mind, unchallenged, you've accepted it as true. Unless you've had reason or evidence otherwise to challenge it, you've taken that belief on as your own. That thought will remain in your mind, even if it's pushed into your subconscious where you might be unaware of it, until something or someone triggers it, and you react to it emotionally without really knowing why.

In order to better understand our thoughts, it's important to know how they work. Imagine our mind as having two levels to it, like a house for instance, with the main floor being the conscious mind and the basement being the subconscious. This analogy allows us to see how there are two parts of our mind, working together, existing "under the same roof": the **conscious** and the **subconscious**.

The conscious part of our mind is responsible for logic and reasoning. For instance, if you were asked to count the peas on your plate, it's your conscious mind that will add it up. The conscious mind also controls your voluntary actions, so when you decide to move your arms or legs, it's your conscious mind telling you to carry out the action.

The subconscious part of your mind is responsible for all of your involuntary actions. Your breathing and heartbeat are controlled by your subconscious. You don't have to think about it or tell your heart to beat because it's doing it on its own—it's automatic. Think of it like driving a car. When you first learned to drive, you had to really focus and concentrate. But the more you did it, the more familiar and comfortable you became on the road, and the less you had to "think" about what you needed to do. It became automatic because your subconscious absorbed how to drive from you on a conscious level. You were feeding your subconscious information like, "A red light means stop. Green means go." Once we became proficient at driving, we no longer had to consciously process what we did when we came to a red light; our subconscious took over and our reaction was automatic. The information was stored in our memory—our subconscious.

We teach our subconscious everything it knows, meaning we're constantly feeding it information—and that doesn't just mean the correct way to drive a car. It means we also feed it information that can also **not** be positive or productive to our well-being. In other words, our thoughts are not as cut and dry as what to do at a red light; that is, we may not necessarily think we're telling ourselves things that aren't good for us when we're thinking and processing thoughts that are invalidating or detrimental, any more than we would tell ourselves to speed through a red light. However, if we believe our thoughts to be true without challenging them, we run the risk of storing them in our subconscious as our reality, whether they are true and real or not, and that can be threatening or dangerous to our well-being too.

Why wouldn't we put the same care and attention that we put into learning to drive a car as we do into what we tell ourselves? It's imperative to question our negative thoughts as soon as they pop up in our conscious mind in order to catch them and challenge them before they get stored in our subconscious as beliefs.

It's important to also note that while the subconscious mind is the basement/storage area for our thoughts, it is also responsible for the automatically triggered feelings and emotions that we suddenly experience upon facing each situation. Until we know what thoughts our conscious mind is telling our subconscious, we are not in control of what we think we are—which can affect every decision we make, every desire we have, every goal we want to realize. More than just facilitating our feelings, which dictate our actions, the conscious and subconscious are our entire thoughts *combined*, which is a pretty powerful combination.

## Conscious vs. Subconscious Thoughts

Napoleon Hill, the 20th century pioneer of positive thinking, once observed that, "The subconscious mind makes no distinction between constructive and destructive thought impulses; (it) will translate into reality a thought driven by fear, just as readily as it will translate into reality a thought driven by courage or faith." That's why it is up to us to discern the difference.

And the only way we can "discern" the difference between "constructive and destructive" thoughts is to question them to find out which ones serve our well-being, and which ones don't. If they are derived from a distorted perception we have of something we've experienced, or have been influenced by a negative opinion or belief of someone else, then they will cause our thoughts to be "driven by fear", and will not serve our well-being. Sticking with the basement analogy, that the subconscious is like a the storage room of all of your memories from the experiences you've had, both positive and negative, it's not until we delve deeper into our subconscious to find out what beliefs are stored there that we can begin to weed out what is negative (destructive), and keep what is positive (constructive). Until we do, we will constantly be at the affect of our negative, fear-based thoughts running our minds.

*Questioning your thoughts not only reaches*
*your conscious but subconscious as well.*

When a negative thought pops up in our mind, it usually triggers an emotion, like sadness or anger, and it's only by questioning those thoughts that you can find out why you feel the way you do. By doing so, you delve deeper into what's stored in your subconscious (and why it's there). This is necessary, especially if you need to clear out some of those thoughts and let them go. You aren't just skimming the surface of your thoughts. Finding the source of negative thoughts requires you to go deeper into your "thought base": your subconscious. Unless you reach far in there, you are only putting a band-aid on your negative thoughts—covering them up without addressing the deeper wound. You aren't getting to the bottom of them to find out why they are there in the first place, lurking below the surface and popping up during periods of stress or emotional turbulence.

The conscious mind monitors whatever thoughts arise, and serves as a filter to either accept or reject them. What it chooses to accept or reject has a lot to do with what thoughts seem useful or beneficial for one's sense of "self" or "identity". So if you have a negative opinion of yourself, you will allow for negative thoughts to come in and "stay there," which your subconscious absorbs as your beliefs, and those beliefs will stay real for as long as you allow for them to. If you've accepted as your reality the belief that you're fat based on something someone said to you about your weight a long time ago, and still hold it as true, it remains stored in your subconscious, and whenever you are in a situation where you have to show your body, like on a summer cruise or on the beach in a bathing suit, for example, you may be prone to feeling depressed or anxious without ever connecting it to when that thought was "accepted" as your reality. You will have a "fixed" belief about your body that it's not good enough because someone told that to you, and until you question and challenge it with the *Says Who?* method to find out that it's not your original thought, you will be at the affect of it time and time again.

The same can be said for any negative belief you have and are holding onto. Feelings of inferiority or any kind of self-loathing doesn't just appear out of nowhere. Those negative thoughts that create those feelings are usually tucked away deep in our subconscious, and sometimes are so buried, we are completely unaware that they are hidden within us. It's like walking around with self-hate, and going about your life, even smiling to the world, without ever letting anyone know that there's a part of you that holds yourself in contempt.

Whatever negative thought you tell yourself goes straight into your subconscious and stays there as a belief. The only way a belief can be changed is if you change it on a conscious level, which is done by questioning those beliefs to make sure they are true—that is, whether they are based on fact or simply a "distorted" perception you have.

That's why, whatever you tell yourself, especially if it's negative, your subconscious believes it. And why wouldn't it, since only *you* are the gatekeeper of all your thoughts and beliefs entering into or exiting from your mind. Whatever you accept as real and true, so does your subconscious. Accepting a negative thought like, "I'm fat" or "stupid" or "a failure," will be stored in your subconscious as a belief about yourself. Until you change that thought, your subconscious will keep it as a fixed belief.

For instance, if you tell yourself something like "I'm fat," and want to lose weight, your subconscious registers and accepts that thought as a belief. If you genuinely want to lose weight, "I'm fat," is not the motivating or productive thought you need to be thinking; it's not a useful thought that tells your subconscious what you want to achieve, or what your intention is, but rather it's just name calling and putting yourself down. You're sabotaging yourself even before you start. *If you really want to lose weight, tell yourself you will, and mean it. If you're sincere in your desire, your subconscious will believe you, and hold that belief as true, and together your conscious mind and subconscious mind can work in tandem to achieve the optimum results you want.*

A few years ago supermodel Kate Moss caused quite a furor when she was asked how she was always able to remain model-thin year-in, year-out and she was quoted as saying, "Nothing tastes as good as being skinny feels." Now, you may disagree with her sentiment, but she is an example of someone who is continually reinforcing her desire—to be skinny—to her subconscious. She resists temptation to overindulge in food because she has embedded an image in her mind about how good it looks and feels to be thin.

Your desire and your belief in yourself to realize that desire need to be one and the same, and if they aren't, you will be sending mixed messages to your subconscious, which will store those mixed messages as your beliefs, and that's the very thing you want to avoid. The ultimate goal is to have all of your thoughts and beliefs, conscious and subconscious to be similar and in synch so they can support what you want with clear-minded intention. When we are conflicted, it's important to sort out our thoughts to determine the source of the mixed feelings we are having. Questioning our thoughts is a useful tool in sorting out our thoughts. Doing so helps us identify and recognize the conflicted and contradictory thoughts we are having, such as, "I want to lose weight, but I'm afraid I won't be able to do it." It's okay and even common to have a thought like that, which combines a positive intention with a doubt or fear. But keep in mind that the thought that will best set your desire in motion is, "I want to lose weight." That's the one you want to focus on and repeat like a mantra because, remember, your subconscious is listening! The second part of the thought, "but I'm afraid I won't be able to do it" supports fear and doubt, and that is the part you need to question and challenge.

It's also important to make sure that whatever it is we desire to do, it's backed up and supported with positive, affirmative thoughts. Just having the desire to do something, like losing weight, is not enough to make it happen. Just ask anyone who's ever made a New Year's resolution! You have to continue your mental discipline by staying focused and vigilant about not letting other thoughts, negative or mixed, be a part of your thinking process when you want to reach a goal.

Say you're trying to quit an addictive habit like smoking. It's one thing to say you want to quit, but it's extremely difficult to be successful, especially since research shows smoking is one of the hardest habits to break. Yes, saying what we want to do is important and a good place to start, but if you light up a cigarette after you've decided to quit and make excuses and tell yourself something like, "I'm just having one after lunch and that's okay," you are clearly sending a mixed message to your subconscious that it *is* okay, and that's *not* going to help you quit at all. That is a perfect example of a desire that is not in synch with a thought.

There are people who smoke who will even say, "It's a disgusting habit, I know," and light right up anyway. Even though they would like nothing more than to quit, if they're saying those kinds of contradictory thoughts to themselves and think such words are meaningless and thus won't interfere with their goal, unfortunately those words and thoughts will. Just like telling yourself "I'm fat," you might *say* smoking is a disgusting habit, but until you are truly disgusted by it, and everything else you think supports your unhappiness and disgust with smoking, then quitting smoking will remain only a desire you hope to realize "someday." Unless you're telling yourself exactly what you want to do productively and actively, which I call an "Action Thought," (Chapter Thirteen) then you won't be able to reach your goal successfully.

*Remember, your conscious thoughts and your subconscious beliefs must be one and the same in order for you to achieve your desire. The best way for that to happen is to question any negative thought you have, and remove it before it gets stored in your subconscious as a belief.*

We have to be careful, also, that we don't set ourselves up to fail with our thinking, which is why it's so important to be clear about our conscious thoughts, and the message they're sending to our subconscious. Sometimes our goals are set so high that we make it almost impossible for ourselves to reach them, one of the reasons those dreaded New Year's resolutions never seem to work out.

Losing weight is a good example to describe the frustration many people feel about not being able to accomplish what they set out to do. Many times the first thing someone will say when they want to lose weight is the number of pounds they want to drop, which is fine, and can be good for goal setting. But the number they attach to their goal to lose weight can become so daunting to them over time, that their thoughts about losing weight start to weaken and their desire and best intentions can't hold up or sustain itself, and they find themselves unable to reach the number they proclaimed they would.

"I'm going to lose fifty pounds!" a client announced with tremendous enthusiasm to me one day. This happens a lot—getting caught up with excitement and announcing a new goal. Her excitement, however, was more about the number and end result than the day-to-day commitment it takes to actually lose the weight. Therefore, as the days continued, her excitement began to wear off, and the thoughts that are needed to support her "desire" to lose weight began to vanish, and the "belief" in herself to lose weight, especially the number of pounds she'd put in her mind, was no longer there. The problem with that type of thinking is that you're not only left with not realizing your goal, as my client was, but you may even resort to name calling, such as, "I'm a loser," which only exacerbates the shame spiral and confirms a negative subconscious belief.

The key is, once the first troubling thought pops up, to question that thought. Ask yourself, "Says who? Who says I'm a loser?" Doing so allows you to examine it and hold it up to the light of day. Unless you question a negative belief you have about yourself or someone else, or something someone has said about you, it becomes a permanent part of your thinking. Remember, your subconscious takes you literally, so if you're going to proclaim a goal like, "I'm going to lose fifty pounds," make sure it's reasonable and you can stick to it. If you have any doubt that you might not be able to, why not just start with telling yourself something like "I'm going to lose some weight." That's perfectly fine and acceptable, and if you do happen to reach your goal of fifty pounds or however many pounds you want to lose, you'll feel that much better about yourself. The problem with being overzealous or over-demanding of yourself, and getting caught up with numbers or statistics in your mind more than the day-to-day commitment to losing weight is that, if you don't reach your goal, you can end up feeling bad about yourself and revert to name calling, such as, "I'm a failure."

Remember, no name calling! Children do that in the sandbox.

## The Origins of Self-Critical Thinking

Many of our beliefs are formed when we are children and adolescents, and become our "core" beliefs, which are the main ideas we have about ourselves, and continue to have as adults. For us to function in a way that feels good or comfortable, we need to maintain positive core beliefs, meaning holding thoughts like, "I'm likable," or "I'm worthwhile," or "I'm a good person," etc. However, given that we also hold negative core beliefs too, and they often don't rear their ugly heads until we're feeling vulnerable, upset, angry, hurt or stressed, that's when they can automatically pop up as counter-productive thoughts in our minds and feel like they have control or power over our thinking.

As children we don't understand how our thoughts become our core beliefs, and we're very susceptible to being influenced by our peers and the adults around us. We also want to be liked and accepted so it's easier to go along with someone else's opinion, even if we don't necessarily agree or like it. So the result is we often grow up with some negativity in our belief system, and it can become rigid or even fixed about certain ideas or opinions we have. It's not until you ask yourself as an adult questions about a negative or fear-based thought you have, which has turned into a belief, that you can think back and remember who it was that told you that you "weren't good enough," or "weren't going to amount to anything," or something that was critical or demeaning that might have been said to you at one time. This helps you connect the dots to when your thinking stopped being authentically your own. By doing this you can then realize that this negative thought you've been carrying around for so long about yourself:

1. Is not your original thought.
2. You've heard it said by someone else.
3. You don't like.
4. Does not make you feel better.
5. Does not work for you.
6. Controls your thinking.
7. You don't want to keep.

A thought that does not serve your well-being or influences your life in a negative way is often a thought that is blown out of proportion—that is, distorted and therefore not real. A thought that is real can be backed up with evidence or fact, and known to be true based on proof. But let's say you can back up a thought with proof like you're a "horrible cook", or you're "bad at sports," or "not good at math," with proof (burned dinners or bad grades, for instance) and feel there's nothing distorted or untrue about what you're not good at. The problem really isn't your shortcomings or inabilities. It's the negative, undermining thoughts that continue to berate you that does the most harm. And that can be much more damaging than the truth itself. I mean, all of us are good at some things and not so good at others. That's life. However, it's the negative perception we have about it and the negative things we tell ourselves concerning it that diminishes us and doesn't serve our well-being. It's also how we interpret either a comment someone makes towards us or what we tell ourselves about the things we perceive as weaknesses that determines what we believe is real and what is not.

For example, thinking you're a loser or unlovable can be a *belief* you hold about yourself that you've accepted because you're not good or successful at something. Instead of accepting that as true or real, you need to challenge those negative labels or name calling of yourself by asking "Says who?" By starting with that first question you are challenging the belief that you have about yourself, which helps you realize that just because you may not be good or successful at a particular thing, it does not make you a loser or unlovable.

## Question—and Challenge—Your Thoughts

*Nobody is born a loser or unlovable. Those are opinions and beliefs we grow into believing about ourselves because of how we interpreted a negative experience we had or something someone said about us.*

"Says who?" is asking yourself, "Who says I'm a loser or unlovable?" "Did I tell myself that I'm a loser or unlovable?" or "Did someone else say that about me?" You need to find that out first before you ask yourself the subsequent six questions of the method. It's important to take responsibility for your negative thoughts, and by doing so, you can understand that any negative thought you have is something only you can change if you want to. And even if your negative thought or opinion about yourself was something you accepted because of someone else's opinion of you, it is still up to you to change it if you don't like it. It is as simple as challenging those thoughts with "Says who?", and then following up with a short series of questions designed to determine if your thoughts are serving your well-being by supporting and affirming your desires and goals.

We can tell ourselves all sorts of things we wish were different about ourselves: "I wish I was taller, thinner, smarter, more creative, more successful," etc. All of us have things about ourselves we wish were different, but it's important to be aware when those thoughts go into negative attack mode over what you wish was different about you. There's a big difference between having a wish or an opinion about yourself that is honest and harmless vs. attaching a negative, diminishing thought to it.

Wishing you were thinner, smarter, more successful, or whatever you might wish for are natural desires to have, and sometimes necessary and helpful for motivating you to achieve what you want. However, unless there are positive, affirming thoughts to surround your desire, those negative, diminishing thoughts will threaten to undermine your desires and goals.

I'm not saying that every single thought we have can be or even should be glowing and complimentary, but since every thought you have influences everything in your life, you may as well decide that you want your internal dialogue to be positive and productive, which can only make you feel good about yourself, and a little bit of self praise certainly can't hurt. Honesty about ourselves is one thing, but tearing yourself down is completely useless, counter-productive, and serves no purpose whatsoever for your well-being.

## Your Authentic Self

The *Says Who?* method will help you get to the bottom of your negative thoughts so you can know what is real and what is not. Think of it as your truth barometer, or your compass pointing to your **authentic self**—the you that was whole and existed in a "true nature" state before your negative thoughts and beliefs influenced and distorted your perception of your real essence, self esteem, and healthy image of yourself. It's time to return to your original, authentic self, and be present in your life as someone who deserves to love and accept yourself for who you really are, and meant to be. And if your goals are to change certain things about yourself you would like to improve, go easy with kindness, and not negative criticism. You will get much more positive results by encouraging yourself to be better at something, or the best that you can be by thinking thoughts that are productive and supportive. Your thoughts should be your cheering squad, not your hecklers.

Be clear about your desire, and the positive conscious thoughts you tell yourself, which then gets stored in your subconscious as beliefs.

However, just getting to know your thoughts and their origin is only the beginning of your journey of awareness, a journey that will allow you to eventually be able to recognize and understand your thoughts better than you ever have before, and let you control them rather than having them control you.

Questioning your thoughts will help you form a productive relationship between you and your thoughts, meaning that it will yield a cohesive working system where your thoughts that are allowed to "occupy" your mind have been cleared by you first. This also holds you accountable for them, an important step if you want to be in charge of your thoughts. You need to be the regulator of what thoughts stay in and what thoughts go out.

However, in order for you to truly be able to put the *Says Who?* method to work and get the best results out of it, it's important to be completely committed to understanding how your thoughts work, and want to change the negative ones into positive productive thoughts with consistency. This needs to become your new way of thinking, which requires a mental discipline. Just like you would exercise to take care of your body and keep it fit and in good shape, or eat well to take care of your health, you need to take care of your thinking, and make sure your mental health is optimum.

## The First Step

Even before you use the *Says Who?* method, the first thing to do when an unpleasant or negative thought comes into your head and threatens to throw you off stride is to **acknowledge** it right away.

*Acknowledge—Recognize its existence, even if it's upsetting. Don't deny it or try to push it away. This allows you to recognize that you are having a negative thought and admit to yourself that it is happening. This keeps you in **the present** moment. Being in the present moment is important because it allows you to focus on what is occurring in the "now," which is actual and real, instead of the emotion surrounding the thought.*

Doing this will help put you in the **observer mode**, instead of **reactive mode**.

*Observer Mode—Observing your thought means you are listening to it like a witness. This allows you to separate yourself from your negative thought and be independent of it. By doing this you are not reacting to it or having it influence your state of mind in any way, but merely aware of it.*

*Reactive Mode—Being reactive is the opposite of observing. Reactive Mode means you are responding to your negative thought quickly without acknowledging or observing it. When you are in this state of mind you cannot separate yourself from your negative thought nor can you question it to find out if it is real or not. You are at the mercy of your negative thought and it is controlling you.*

By *acknowledging* your negative thought, and then examining it closely as an *observer* and not a *reactor*, you can identify whether it is a productive thought that helps you function in a positive way in life and serves your well-being or if it's a thought that makes you feel bad or fearful, and serves no purpose for your well-being at all.

You can then begin the *Says Who?* questioning process to find out what that thought is doing in your mind, and what it wants from you. Think of it as an intruder. The first thing you would want to ask someone who is trespassing or invading your space is, "What are you doing here?" or "What do you want?" They don't belong on your private property, and have no right to be there.

The same can be said about a negative, intrusive thought that pops up in your mind unexpectedly and uninvited. By being the observer you're applying the same kind of questioning to your negative or disruptive thoughts as you would an intruder. That's why the first thing you need to ask yourself when a negative thought pops into your mind is "Says who?" which means, "Who is saying this thought in my mind and why?" This immediately helps establish what it's doing in your mind and what it wants from you. This first question will also start the process needed to challenge and identify your negative thought as real or not real.

The subsequent questions will challenge your negative thought even more so that you can get to the bottom of it and the intention behind it. By probing further you can then decide if you want to keep your negative thought or let it go—a decision that is completely up to you. You are in control of your thoughts, always.

---

By asking a negative thought "Says who?" you are demanding it to reveal who is responsible for this thought in your mind. In other words, how did it get there? Once you find out, then you are responsible for what you want to do about it. Is it your original thought, or was it someone else's and you took it on as your own? You may even discover it is an old thought that has become part of your core beliefs, and now it's time to challenge it and let it go.

---

## Chapter 3

# The *Says Who?* Method

*The mind gives an order to the body and it is at once obeyed,*
*but when it gives an order to itself, it is resisted.*
**—Saint Augustine**

The *Says Who?* questioning method will begin the process needed for you to know and understand your thoughts better, so that you can be prepared to challenge a negative thought when it unexpectedly pops up and wants to undermine, sabotage, control, or keep you from being your authentic self, and reaching your goals to lead a happy and fulfilled life.

As I've said, you cannot lead a happy and fulfilled life if your inner dialogue is conflicted or causing you to suffer. When you commit to using the following questions, and allow them to be your guide for managing your thoughts, you will see how clear and sharp your perception will become, and how you are able to discern and identify quickly which of your thoughts are real and which are not. By using the *Says Who?* method with consistency, the bottom line will eventually be, "If this thought doesn't support my well-being, then I have no use for it."

Using the method regularly will also give you the tools to immediately identify, challenge and resist any negative thought that tries to pull you down a non-productive path. It will enable you to refuse to give in to the type of negative thoughts that can cause you to take a "wrong turn" and derail you from reaching your goals. *Says Who?* will help you stay on course so you can create the positive mindset needed to reach fulfillment.

---

**The *Says Who?* Questions:**
1. Says Who?
2. Have I heard someone say this thought before?
3. Do I like this thought?
4. Does this thought make me feel better?
5. Does this thought work for me?
6. Am I in control of this thought?
7. Do I want to keep this thought or let it go?

---

These seven questions will be the tools in your arsenal to combat what can often feel like a mental battle in our minds. Having them at your disposal whenever you need them will allow you to feel equipped to master your mind at all times. You will feel empowered knowing that you are in control of your thoughts—they are not in control of you!

## Breaking Down the Questions

By asking yourself "Says Who?"—you are confronting and challenging a negative or fear based thought to find out what it's doing in your mind. By answering, "I am saying this thought," you now assume responsibility for your thought, and can begin the process of questioning and examining it more closely to find out what purpose it's serving for your well being. Subsequently, by asking yourself:

*Have I heard someone say this thought before?*—You're finding out if this is your original thought, or if it came into your mind because you heard someone else—such as a parent, relative, teacher, spouse, boss, or anyone other than yourself—say this to you before. By identifying the originator of the thought, you are able to know if it isn't your original thought, and does not belong to you as your own.

*Do I like this thought?*—You're finding out if this thought is desirable or appealing to you. If not, why are you thinking it?

*Does this thought make me feel better?*—You're finding out if this thought builds you up or tears you down; improves how you feel or makes you feel worse. If it doesn't make you feel better about yourself or enhances your self-esteem in any way, why are you thinking it?

*Does this thought work for me?*—You're finding out if this thought is useful or productive for you, and if it supports your desires or goals. If not, why are you thinking it?

*Am I in control of this thought?*—You're finding out if this thought has any kind of hold or power over you, or whether you are in control of it. If not, why you would think a thought that has the power to have control over you?

*Do I want to keep this thought or let it go?*—You're finding out if you want to hold on to a thought that serves no useful purpose for your well-being, If not, are you willing to let it go?

So, unless you know the answers to these questions:

- Is it your own original thought?
- Is it someone else's thought?
- Do you like this thought?
- Does this thought make you feel better?
- Does this thought work for you?
- Are you in control of your thought?
- Do you want to keep this thought or let it go?

......**you do not know your thoughts entirely.**

The next several chapters, which investigate the types of thoughts we have, are designed to give you a crash course in helping you identify and recognize your thoughts and certain patterns of thinking that lead to emotional land mines and derailing you from your purpose.

## Chapter 4
# Fear Based Thoughts

*Fear is only as deep as the mind allows.*
**—Japanese Proverb**

Fear is an emotion we feel when we think our survival is being threatened. We usually feel it when we experience pain or when we sense danger. It's an important instinct to have, and it helps us recognize something that can be harmful to us so we can protect ourselves or flee from it if we have to. When we're frightened, we experience it in our body as a "fight or flight" response. Our heart beats fast, our palms get sweaty, and our thinking goes into alert or panic mode: "I'm in danger!" or "Get the hell out of here!" or "I'm going to die!" Fear is an important basic survival mechanism to protect us.

Fear-based thoughts, on the other hand, can have the opposite effect. The difference between fear of a genuine threat and a fear-based thought is that fear-based thoughts have no basis in protecting our survival from something that is truly harmful or life-threatening. They are simply worries, doubts and/or insecurities, which often are exaggerated, blown out of proportion, and can even be imagined or not true. Those types of fear-based thoughts need to be challenged as to why they make us feel we are truly in actual danger when we're not. They shouldn't dominate or hold us captive, unless again, we're in some kind of genuine danger.

An example would be fear of flying. Many people are terrified to get on a plane for fear it will crash. It doesn't matter how many statistics you quote to them about how flying is an infinitely more safe way to travel than driving. The fear of crashing overwhelms any statement of fact. That fear will stay "fixed" in their mind as a belief, and the only way that can change is to question and challenge it, then replace it with a new belief that if they get on a plane, it will not crash.

That's not to say that if you get on a plane, you won't feel nervous or frightened ever again. If you have a genuine fear of flying, you may never feel totally secure or comfortable on a plane, but you can learn to manage, and even control the kinds of fear-based thoughts that can paralyze you.

So how do you shed light on fear, and see it for what it really is? You question it by asking, "Says who?" Like a boogieman in your mind, you need to stand up to it and let it know who's in control and the boss of your thoughts. It's either you or your fear-based thought. It's important to decide who's really in charge of your thinking.

Depending on how you've interpreted an unpleasant, traumatic, or life-threatening event in your life, fear can play a very important role in how you feel or think about anything that appears, resembles or mimics a similar threat or danger to your survival. In other words, if something happened to you that was frightening—for example, you encountered a snake while you were hiking, and you processed it in your mind by telling yourself something like "I'm not safe when I'm hiking," you will hold that belief in your mind every time you go for a hike. Or, you may decide to give up hiking altogether on the off chance you might run into another snake. That's an example of when a fear-based thought can stop or paralyze you, keeping you from doing something you really want to do. It's another illustration of when your desires are not in synch with your thoughts. If what you wish for cannot be supported by positive and encouraging thoughts, then you cannot actualize those desires, and they frustratingly remain only a longing instead of reality.

Being aware that snakes are nearby is important, cautious and wise, but if that thought stops you from doing what you want to do in your life, like hiking, or doesn't allow you to enjoy it while you're doing it, then that is what happens when a fear-based thought dominates your thinking so much so you can't let it go.

Sometimes our fears aren't even based on something as tangible as a snake. Many of us fear new experiences, taking risks or exposing ourselves to ridicule. This is evidenced by that age-old survey that shows that more people fear public speaking than death. This is an obvious demonstration of how a fear-based thought can keep someone from doing something they are convinced will cause them public humiliation. "Why am I so successful?" the legendary Dolly Parton once said. "I worked without fear. So that gave me freedom."

Holding onto fearful thoughts can interfere with the quality of your life on many levels. Snakes are a universal fear that a lot of people have, but that doesn't mean that it stops everyone from being out in nature or enjoying hiking. Some people don't think about it while they're walking or hiking in an area where snakes are, and view it as something they'll deal with if or when it happens.

It's what you do with your fears, and how you handle them that determine the choices you make and how you live your life, and whether or not you enjoy the things you want to do, or can achieve the goals or success you desire. If you're someone who genuinely likes to hike, and have encountered a snake which frightened you to the point where it's put you off to hiking and you have thoughts such as, "I'm not safe when I'm hiking," you have the choice to question and challenge that thought by using the *Says Who?* method. By asking yourself, "Does this thought work for me?" you can see how your thought isn't working for you favorably because it's stopping you from doing something you really enjoy.

Everyone has something that frightens them, whether it's snakes, spiders, public speaking, a fear of heights, etc., but again, it's how much you let your fears interfere with what you want to do that matters. The thoughts you tell yourself that surround your fears are what determines whether you will succumb to them, and perhaps even be paralyzed by them, or overcome them.

## Challenging the Source of Fear-Based Thoughts

Sometimes our fears aren't so easy to identify, like snakes or spiders, and they're buried deeper within us. For example, a fear could be related to an incident that happened early on in your life that involved something like abandonment or distrust, such as when a family is broken up when a parent leaves the home, never to return, through divorce or death. Or it can be the death of another loved one. Again, depending on how an upset or trauma is interpreted and processed in your mind, it makes a significant difference in how you perceive anything that happens in the future that appears, resembles or mimics that similar feeling you had when you first experienced that original disruption or devastation.

We've all experienced troubles and some kind of loss in our formative years—it's part of growing up. However, as I said in Chapter Two when discussing the subconscious, it's what you think and tell yourself about those experiences that you accept as real, that becomes a belief. For example, if you experienced abandonment through divorce early in your life, and thought something like, "People abandon you when you get close to them," or "Marriage doesn't work," or "I'll never be vulnerable to someone else because they can hurt me," unless you challenge those beliefs, you will continue to hold them as real and true, and they can be what perpetuates your fear and fear-based thoughts about love, intimacy or marriage.

In my life coaching practice I've worked with people who have very strong opinions and beliefs about things they experienced in their childhood, and made decisions and choices in their life because of how those events affected them. For instance, I had a client who grew up with parents she believed didn't really love each other, and made a decision to never get married because she feared that marriage can poison and ruin a relationship. Even though she has been in a relationship for over twenty years, and genuinely loves her partner, her association to marriage is a negative and fear-based one because of how she perceived and interpreted her parents' relationship. Her partner has asked her repeatedly to marry him, but she will not take that next step, preferring instead to keep "well enough alone" in order to not, in her perspective and with no real evidence, ruin the relationship—a perfect example of how a stored belief, which may not even originate with you, can alter your reality and even hinder your quality of life.

That is why asking yourself, "Have I heard someone say this thought before," you might realize that you heard someone from your past say a thought you currently hold true, like, "Marriage doesn't work," and you took that belief on as your own. And even if that thought is your original thought because of how you perceived a negative situation, you still have the choice to question your thoughts and beliefs so you can decide if they are working for you, *and if you want to let them go.*

In experiencing situations such as the fear of marriage or abandonment, you can spend your whole life trying to avoid being in a similar situation that makes you feel vulnerable to another person, or you can decide to confront your thoughts and beliefs about abandonment by challenging them, using the following *Says Who?* method. I'm using the example of "People abandon you when you get close to them," but you can substitute it with any fear-based thoughts you want:

*Says who?*

**Which means**: "Who is saying that people abandon you when you get close to them? Is this something I am telling myself because I believe it?"

**Your answer might be**: "I am telling myself that people can abandon you when you get close to them. Why do I believe that?"

*Have I heard someone say this thought before?*

**Which means**: "Can I recall hearing someone say that people abandon you when you get close to them?"

**Your answer might be**: "I remember someone telling me when I was growing up that people can abandon you when you get close to them and I believed them. Why do I still believe what they told me?"

*Do I like this thought?*

**Which means**: "Do I like thinking that people abandon you if you get close to them?"

**Your answer can be**: "No, I don't like thinking that people can abandon me if I get close to them, so why am I thinking a thought I don't like?"

*Does this thought make me feel better?*

**Which means**: "Does thinking that people abandon you when you get close to them make me feel better about myself?"

**Your answer can be**: "Thinking that people can abandon me if I get close to them doesn't make me feel better at all. It makes me feel insecure and doubtful of others and I can choose not to think a thought that doesn't make me feel good."

*Does this thought work for me?*

**Which means**: "Does thinking that people abandon you if you get close to them serve my well-being?"

**Your answer can be**: "Thinking that people can abandon me if I get close to them makes me feel distrustful, and that doesn't work favorably for me or serve my well-being."

*Am I in control of this thought?*

**Which means**: "Does thinking that people abandon you if you get close to them control or dominate my thoughts?"

**Your answer can be**: "Thinking that people can abandon me if I get close to them dominates my thoughts when I care for someone or feel vulnerable to them. I don't want to be controlled by a thought that is full of fear."

*Do I want to keep this thought or let it go?*

**Which means**: "Do I want to keep thinking that people abandon you when you get close to them, or release it?"

**Your answer can be**: "Thinking that people can abandon me if I get close to them is not a thought I want to hold onto, **and I choose to let it go**."

Fear-based thoughts keep our fears alive and very real for us. Unless we want to keep those thoughts as our "fixed" beliefs, meaning that they aren't going anywhere, we need to change them by questioning and challenging them to find out if they are serving our well being. *Says Who?* is the very method that will accomplish that. Even though you might not feel an instant release of your fears or see them vanish overnight the first time you challenge them, over time, a consistency of questioning your thoughts with the method will create something akin to a muscle memory; that is, your beliefs regarding your fears will begin to change, and you will find they no longer have a grip or hold on you. You will start to feel a shift in your whole thinking process, which is empowering. In fact, you will probably wonder why you tolerated some of those negative thoughts you had for so long!

It certainly happened for me when I realized I didn't have to live in fear that I could have a nervous breakdown like my sister. By changing my fear-based thoughts, I took responsibility for them, which allowed me to take control over them and create the life I wanted.

By questioning your fears, you can find out if they are actually real and based in fact, or a result of how you perceived a negative experience you've had and then turned it into a belief. *If you want to change a fear-based belief, then you need to change the thoughts that support it.*

Questioning your thoughts with the *Says Who?* method will not only change any thoughts that support negativity and fear, but it will keep you in the here and now, in the present. It will force you to look at what you're thinking in the very moment you're thinking it. If your thoughts are fear-based, the questions will challenge them right then and there, and immediately help you change the negative thoughts around them so they don't escalate into something like anxiety, or even panic. The method helps release the fearful thoughts that have a hold on you—like avoiding hiking because of snakes, or resisting marriage because of fear of a negative outcome, or avoiding intimacy because of the possibility of abandonment, and replacing them with positive, fearless thoughts that make you feel there's nothing you can't do or overcome!

If you want to stay centered and empowered in your life, you must be willing to question and challenge your negative and fear-based thoughts whenever they come up. Do not wait to challenge them because they will only grow stronger in your mind and keep a hold on you!

By drawing upon your strength from within, and doing the daily mental work it takes to have and *keep* a healthy sense of self, you will begin to see and feel a significant difference in your life, like feeling less fear, having more confidence, and more inner peace. If we don't take the necessary steps to support and nurture our inner core, then we will forever be at the mercy of external influences and circumstances that will decide whether we feel good about ourselves, instead of ourselves making that decision.

Develop that inner strength first—through a daily practice of questioning your thoughts—and everything else will support it, not deplete it.

# Chapter 5
# Automatic Thoughts

*A mind too active is no mind at all.*
**—Theodore Roethke**

Wouldn't it be great if we could somehow predict when a negative thought was going to enter our mind? Then we could head it off at the pass and challenge it, all without interrupting our day or causing it to perpetuate itself. However, we know that's not realistic, because, as we've learned, that's not how thoughts work. Our mind is so busy with thoughts coming and going all day that regulating them seems almost impossible. That's because our thoughts are often **Automatic Thoughts**.

Automatic thoughts are what most of the thoughts that we have in any given situation are called. They're referred to as "automatic" because we don't ask for them to pop up in our minds—they just do. They are involuntary, not pre-meditated, and can happen when we least expect it, during the most unlikely or unexpected situations, because something or someone has triggered a reaction or response in us that resulted in this automatic thought.

An example: when someone cuts you off in traffic. An automatic thought that might immediately pop up in your mind could be, "What an idiot!" and you may even be compelled to yell or gesture at them in protest and anger. This is a knee-jerk response to something someone has done that's upset you and it's directly the result of Automatic Thinking.

Because automatic thoughts can pop up so quickly, and sometimes what we think or say in response is so sudden, we can surprise ourselves by our reaction. How often have we heard someone else blurt something out in the heat of the moment that can be embarrassing, insulting, or even shocking? That's a result of their automatic thinking.

While I emphasized in Chapter Three the importance of starting your questioning process in the observer mode rather than reactive mode, when an automatic thought pops up because you're reacting to something quickly and are thrown off guard, you probably haven't even had the chance to observe it, let alone question it.

It's usually those types of unexpected situations we find ourselves in—like being cut off in traffic, or if someone is rude or disrespectful to us—when an automatic thought reveals exactly what we're feeling in that moment. It could be hurt, anger, or even hate, and if we don't question our reaction to our automatic thought in the aftermath, it can bring on more negative thoughts, one right after the other, in quick succession, and before we know it our entire thinking has been commandeered by one negative automatic thought that has taken over our entire mood and state of mind. What started off as a good day or a pleasant experience can change in a matter of seconds.

Thinking that someone is an idiot because they cut you off in traffic might be a very justifiable thought for you, but sometimes what can happen is that negative automatic thought doesn't stop there; the next thing you know your heart starts pounding and your adrenaline gets pumping, and suddenly you're involved in a dangerous game of road rage because of a thought gone wild.

The type of anger that can cause someone to engage in road rage isn't something that just erupts out of nowhere because someone cut you off in traffic and pissed you off. It's an emotion connected to a particular belief that's lying beneath the surface, which can rear its ugly head when something unexpected happens, and provokes that belief. In other words, if you hold the belief that aggressive drivers are a menace to society and it's your job to straighten them out, or someone who is rude to you doesn't respect you or has it in for you, your anger will go off because of an external incident that you've allowed to trigger it.

That's why when thoughts go unchecked or unquestioned, especially if it's a knee-jerk type of automatic negative thought that makes you feel agitated or angry (and can escalate into an argument or fight with someone), it's important to catch it as fast as you can—even if it's after the fact—and try to ask yourself any of the *Says Who?* questions.

Here's how the method would work with the thought, "Aggressive drivers are a menace to society, and I've got to go after them and straighten them out":

1. Says who?
   *Who is saying this thought that I must go after this person? Is this something I'm telling myself to do?*
2. Have I heard someone say this thought before?
   *Where have I heard or gotten the thought that aggressive drivers are a menace to society and it's my job to straighten them out?*
3. Do I like this thought?
   *Do I like these types of negative, hair-trigger thoughts that cause me to make snap judgments of others?*
4. Does this thought make me feel better?

*Does this over-reactive type of thinking empower me or make me feel good about myself?*

5. Does this thought work for me?

   *What is this thought doing for me? Is it helping me in any way, or improving my quality of life?*

6. Am I in control of this thought?

   *I seem to be taken over by my anger at this person and not in control of this thought; is that how I want to be?*

7. Do I want to keep this thought or let it go?

   *Do I want to keep thinking about what an idiotic, rude person it is that cut me off and obsess over it, or should I let it go?*

This questioning method will immediately help you center yourself so that you won't be at the affect of a negative, automatic thought that can easily lead you to react to it. Automatic thoughts often can be far too tempting not to respond to. It's like getting pushed or poked—causing a knee-jerk reaction. The whole purpose of questioning a charged automatic thought is to **take charge of it,** and begin the process of controlling it instead of reacting to it.

Asking yourself, "Does this thought work for me?" or, "Am I in control of this thought?" or, "Do I want to keep this thought or let it go?" are perfect questions to ask yourself if you find that your automatic thought is starting to spin out of control and take you further into **reactive mode,** which could be something like road rage. Remember, reactive mode means you are responding to a negative thought quickly without acknowledging or observing it. When you are in this state of mind you cannot separate yourself from your negative thought nor can you question it to find out if it is real or not. You are at the mercy of your negative thought and it is controlling you.

If you find yourself going to a place in your thoughts that is completely counter-productive to your well-being (or perhaps someone else's), nip it in the bud as fast as you possibly can by asking yourself as many of the *Says Who?* questions you are able to. You'll find that even the process of stopping yourself to observe and ask the questions— kind of like the old "Count to Ten" axiom—helps steer the thought and situation towards a calmer, more reflective state of mind.

Thinking someone is an idiot because they cut you off might be exactly what you feel about them in the moment, but again, *if a thought like that, or any thought that stays emotional or heated for you doesn't lighten up quickly and dissolve, then you are not in control of it, and are choosing not to let it go.* Remember, you always have a choice with your negative thoughts—to either keep them or let them go.

There is nothing productive or useful about holding onto a thought that is fueled by anger. It will just keep you angry, and even if you push that anger down, the next time a similar incident happens that upsets you, you're back to the same cycle of automatic negative thinking, which is like being on a hamster wheel of rage and resentment you can't get off.

Even if you have a reactive thought like "What an idiot!" if someone cuts you off in traffic, you can't turn back time and roll the words back into your mouth, but you *can* still go into observer mode right after that thought and ask yourself, "Does this thought make me feel better?" or "Does this thought work for me?" or "Do I want to keep this thought or let it go?" Asking yourself any one of these questions will quickly help you realize that you don't want to waste your good energy on this and move on. It will also force you to confront those triggers that cause you to experience those types of automatic thoughts in the first place. If you discover, from the questioning process, the source of what triggers your knee-jerk response—say, your likening a stranger's cutting you off with your overall sense that no one respects you—you will eventually train your mind to become aware of those triggers and deal with them, meaning your reactions will be less automatic going forward. The process allows you to inspect these triggers and look to see if there is something deeper going on that needs to be examined. Automatic thoughts can actually be very useful if we look at what they evoke in us, and if we can remain the *observer* rather than the *reactor*, we can get to what's most valuable beneath the automatic thought.

In other words, by questioning a thought like, "Aggressive drivers are a menace to society and it's my job to straighten them out," ask yourself, "Have I heard someone else say this thought before?" You might suddenly remember that you grew up with a father who was always yelling at people when he was driving, and realize that you're behaving just like him! Those realizations or epiphanies can be life changing for us (again, the "aha" moment), and the best way to bring that realization about is by being willing to question our automatic thoughts, especially the things that make us hair-trigger mad or cause us to react (or over-react).

*Remember, all of our beliefs are stored in our subconscious, so if an automatic thought triggers a belief that may or may not be originally your own, and it goes unquestioned, unchallenged or unchanged, it will remain there as a belief, prone to being triggered again and again by any random external event that occurs.*

Yes, it's annoying to have someone cut you off in traffic, but it doesn't necessarily mean that the reason they did it has anything to do with your belief that they're a menace to society or they have it in for you, etc. It could simply be that they're just a bad, careless driver, and what you might want to do is get out of their way and not over-analyze it.

If you have automatic thoughts you can't seem to let go of around something someone does or says to you, stick to questioning them with the *Says Who?* method over and over again if you have to. Eventually, one of the questions will awaken something within you, even if it's to help you remember something negative that happened to you in your past that you've stored away in your subconscious as a belief. Maybe the reason you can't shake off the automatic thought you're having is because it's time for you to finally get to the bottom of it to find out why it pops up in your mind when something triggers it. It could be that you're finally ready to let that belief go, and by doing so, you'll notice that the thoughts around that belief will begin to dissolve. How freeing!

Automatic thoughts will always be a part of your thinking, but by understanding them better by questioning them with the *Says Who?* method, you won't allow yourself to be pulled along with them, nor react to them as they come and go in and out of your mind.

# Chapter 6
# Judgmental Thoughts

*If you judge, investigate.*
**—Seneca**

J ust like someone cutting you off in traffic can trigger an automatic thought like, "What an idiot!" (or something with more expletives), sometimes we don't need something rude or aggressive to occur to evoke a thought or reaction in us that can be surprising or throw us off guard.

You can walk into a party, a business meeting, or any social situation, and find yourself having a visceral feeling about someone you've never met before, and a negative or judgmental thought about them suddenly pops into your mind. It could be, "This person is dull or boring," or, "They're pretentious or a snob," or, "They're unattractive," or even, "They're *too* attractive." I could go on and on with the type of thoughts we have about others (and some of them can be really nasty), but I think you get the idea.

We make snap judgments about people without knowing them based on how they look, act, or even how they speak. But how we perceive someone, especially if it's immediately upon seeing or meeting them for the first time, may be directly linked or connected to our beliefs, which, as we now know, affects our thoughts and our behavior. Based on what those beliefs are, they can influence or distort our perception about someone we barely even know. That's not to say that someone can't be off-putting or offensive in their behavior when we meet them, and no matter what our beliefs are, they just rub us the wrong way, and we don't feel drawn to them, period. If you can subscribe to the Buddha quote "Recognize others as yourself," then maybe you can be more forgiving or tolerant of others shortcomings or inadequacies, but not everyone chooses to see others as possessing aspects of themselves, as unattractive as that may be.

Sometimes we need to use discernment rather than harsh judgment when it comes to identifying certain characteristics in someone, and if they're undesirable or distasteful to you, and you don't happen to agree with Buddha's sentiments, recognize how you feel and move on. Not everyone has to be each other's cup of tea. But sometimes you've made up your mind about someone a little too quickly, and if they aren't offensive or off putting as far as you (or others) can see, you might want to look a little further as to why you feel judgmental, and quick to dismiss them.

Our thoughts are largely made up of opinions, values and judgments. How we see ourselves, and others, is entirely based on what we believe, and our beliefs are formed early on in our lives as a result of the experiences we've had, positive or negative. How others have influenced us also affects our experiences and how we come to know things, which also helps shape who we are, and can sway our beliefs.

As adults we're pretty set in our beliefs and accept them as real for us, which I've explained become our core beliefs—that is, the main ideas we have about ourselves and others. The good news is that we live in a free country, and nobody can tell us what to believe or what not to, but that doesn't necessarily mean that we are always accepting or tolerant of each other's beliefs, which can be the reason why we are judgmental of others because of our differences. Politics is always a hot topic when it comes to people's differences, and if you and your friends have different political views, you know it's probably a good idea not to discuss them over dinner, unless you're prepared to get into a heated debate or argument, which, if not handled respectfully, can spoil a good evening if you let it, and possibly even a friendship.

But judging others quickly without really knowing them well is important to pay attention to because you might find something out about yourself that can be both revealing and valuable, and help you get to know yourself better. For some people, their reason for being judgmental of someone can simply be for superficial reasons, like how they're dressed or even wear their hair. But judging someone because of the way they look can be shallow or narrow-minded, and by challenging those thoughts through the *Says Who?* method, you might find out that you're a superficial person, and maybe want to consider changing that about your character because, deep down, you're not proud of that.

Just like asking yourself the *Says Who?* questions about your negative thoughts to find out why they're in your mind and if they're real or not, using the method to investigate your **judgmental thoughts** will also connect you directly to your beliefs, which are what's controlling your thoughts. It's a good opportunity to find out what you're carrying around in the judgmental beliefs department.

Let's say you walk into that party or meeting, and see someone and immediately think to yourself, "I don't like this person." As I outlined in the previous chapter about Automatic Thoughts, the first thing you want to do is "*acknowledge*" your thought, go into "*observer* mode," and not "*reactive* mode," which will help you get to the valuable, underlying information (such as the source of your judgmental beliefs.) Try to identify the emotion around that thought. Remember—they're connected. A thought usually comes up first followed by an emotion, but sometimes you feel something in your gut first, and aren't really sure why. It could be dislike, intimidation, or even jealousy. Again, acknowledge what you're thinking or feeling, observe it without reacting, and then ask yourself the *Says Who?* questions:

| Here's how to apply the method to the thought, "I don't like this person." | |
|---|---|
| **Question:** | **Which can mean:** |
| Says who? | Who is saying "I don't like this person?" Is it me, and if so, why don't I like them? |
| Have I heard someone say this thought before? | Has anyone ever influenced me not to like someone like this person (such as race, religion, looks, mannerisms, etc.), and if so, why am I judging this person based on someone else's beliefs? |
| Do I like this thought? | Do I like holding the thought that I don't like this person based on my judgment of them, and if so, why do I want this thought in my mind? |

| Does this thought make me feel better? | Does thinking that I don't like this person make me feel better about myself, and if so, why do I need to think this thought to feel better about myself? |
|---|---|
| Does this thought work for me? | Does thinking that I don't like this person work for me in a positive way or benefit me somehow, and if so, how? |
| Am I in control of this thought? | Does thinking that I don't like this person control my thoughts right now, or am I in control of this thought, and if I'm in control of it, how, and if not, how? |
| Do I want to keep this thought or let it go? | Do I want to keep thinking that I don't like this person, or do I want to let it go, and if I don't, why not? |

By breaking down the *Says Who?* questions like this and applying them to whatever judgmental thoughts you are thinking, it will help you investigate why a particular thought has come up for you that might need to be looked at more closely. It gives you the tools to delve deeper to get to the "real" reason behind it.

Judgment based on prejudice is a big, and unfortunately, far too common reason why people don't like or accept someone right away. It could be because of that person's religion, or because they're gay that you might be immediately judgmental of them, and whether or not you want to admit that to yourself or not is up to you, but if you are judgmental for those reasons, I would highly suggest asking yourself the

*Says Who?* question, "Have I heard someone say this thought before?" You might be amazed to find out that your judgment comes from something you internalized from someone else—perhaps a parent, sibling, relative, clergy, teacher, etc.—and you've taken their belief on as your own. Prejudice and hate goes back a long way, and we may never be able to pinpoint to where it first began—the original, "Says who?" source—but we certainly can break the chain of perpetuating those hateful beliefs in ourselves.

The only way we can learn to be more tolerant and accepting of others is by questioning our beliefs, and by finding out why they *became* our beliefs in the first place can be very instrumental in letting them go. I've had clients who have asked themselves the question "Have I heard someone say this thought before?" and discovered that they've taken on very strong, and even prejudiced beliefs that were once those of their parents or ex spouse, and are horrified to know they now have them too. Sometimes the minute you make the connection between what your belief is and who influenced it, you can't wait to drop it! I also find it interesting (and sometimes funny) when I hear women say they caught themselves saying something to their children that is exactly what their mothers used to say to them ("I sound just like my mother!"). That's how easy we can be influenced by what someone else has said to us without even knowing it.

It's important not to be passive or lazy about our thoughts, especially judgmental ones. Accepting our judgmental thoughts just because we're thinking them, and not finding out the deeper reasons why, is being passive and lazy, which can lead to ignorance and even arrogance. Thinking you're better than someone without investigating thoroughly why you feel entitled to think that way, or assuming that you're superior to someone because it's your belief that you are above others, is the very thing that separates us from one another, and can foster feelings of elitism, prejudice, and hate. Becoming more aware of your judgmental thoughts by questioning them with the *Says Who?* method can help you embrace others for who they are, rather than rejecting them for what they aren't in your eyes, or what you believe they're not. It all comes down to what you believe, which creates your current thoughts, causing you to judge.

Judgmental thoughts are as easily turned on ourselves as well as others. Thinking that certain things, characteristics or aspects about yourself are good or bad, and right or wrong are associated with judgmental thoughts. Instead of being kind and accepting of yourself, including the things you might view as your weaknesses, you are quick to condemn yourself for your shortcomings instead of supporting and encouraging yourself to be better or the best that you can be. Remember the old adage that there is always someone better off than you as well as someone worse? Well, if you are basing your judgments of people on their economic status, for instance, you may find yourself judging yourself the same way: that is, always striving to "keep up with the Joneses." That's a hamster wheel that never stops—there's always going to be some Jones out there with more than you. Judging yourself by what you don't have in comparison to them is the ultimate self-defeating exercise; the classic no-win situation.

*Says Who?* can help you determine, "Who is telling me that I'm good or bad, or right or wrong, better (richer, smarter) than them or worse?" You need to find out the origin of that thought to know if it's you. Are you judging yourself because of your beliefs, and if so, are those beliefs yours or did someone influence them? That is why asking yourself "Have I heard someone say this thought before?" helps you know if you're carrying around someone else's beliefs that you've taken on as your own.

| How to apply *Says Who?* to a judgmental thought like "I'm not good enough." | |
|---|---|
| **Question:** | **Which can mean:** |
| Says who? | Who is saying I'm not good enough? Is it me, and if so, why do I think I'm not? |
| Have I heard someone say this thought before? | Have I heard someone tell me that I'm not good enough, and if so, why did I believe them? |
| Do I like this thought? | Do I like thinking that I'm not good enough, and if not, why am I thinking it? |
| Does this thought make me feel better? | Does thinking that I'm not good enough make me feel better about myself, and if it doesn't, why am I thinking it? |
| Does this thought work for me? | Does thinking that I'm not good enough work for me, and if it doesn't, why am I thinking it? |
| Am I in control of this thought? | Am I in control of thinking that I'm not good enough, and if so, how, and if not, how? |
| Do I want to keep this thought or let it go? | Do I want to keep thinking that I'm not good enough or let it go, and if I don't, why? |

Other examples of judgmental thoughts people sometimes have about themselves, which result in a negative belief:

1. I'm not (smart, attractive, rich, strong, talented, athletic, etc.) enough. I'm inferior.
2. I've failed at relationships. I'm hopeless.
3. I haven't been successful at anything yet. I'm worthless.
4. I'm overweight. I'm undesirable.
5. I'm not well educated. I'm unintelligent.
6. I come from a poor family. I'm low-class.
7. I'm not creative. I'm boring.
8. Most people my age have accomplished more than I have. I'm hopeless.
9. I'm not good at many things. I'm inept.
10. I can't stick to a diet. I'm pathetic.
11. I never finish what I start. I'm a quitter.
12. All my friends are already married. I'm odd.
13. I give in too easily to others. I'm weak.
14. Others have much more than me. I'm undeserving.

These are just a few of the many examples of the kinds of judgmental thoughts people tell themselves. Some of them can be very undermining and demeaning. Judgmental thoughts like the ones listed above can be a part of your core belief system, and have influenced your thinking and how you feel about yourself for a very long time. Whatever the judgmental thought, whether any of these I mentioned or one of your own, you can plug it into the *Says Who?* method to find the root of the thought and/or belief and that will begin the process of change.

If you've never questioned your judgmental thoughts or beliefs about yourself, then how can you ever change them or believe that change is possible? The *Says Who?* method will put you on the right track to investigate and challenge your negative judgmental beliefs about yourself and/or others. No matter how old you are, where you are, or what you're doing in your life, you can always change those negative beliefs to "believing in yourself" so you can create and have what you want and deserve in your life. But how can you feel deserving if your beliefs tell you that you're not?

*Being judgmental of ourselves is usually connected to expectation.*

We all have things that we ask or require of ourselves, and may aspire to be better people or better at something that we do, which is fine. But in so doing we can run the risk of imposing a too-high standard of excellence on ourselves that might not be realistic—and if we don't reach that ideal expectation, we tell ourselves that we are not good enough or maybe even a bad person. For some people their expectation is to be perfect, which is an impossible ideal. To try and live up to being "beyond improvement" or "flawless" is a terrible burden to place on oneself, not to mention a thought process designed to set yourself up to be disappointed or fail on some level.

Having high expectations of yourself, as I said, is fine, but be aware of the thoughts that surround your expectations. Are they realistic and supportive of what you are capable of, or are they negative, critical and judgmental, and no matter what you do it will never be good enough, and if that's the case, good enough for who?

*Says Who?* asks that question straight on. What it means is, "Who says I'm not good enough or never will be?" And if it's perfection that you're seeking, ask yourself, "Who is telling me to be perfect? Is it me, or did someone once tell me I have to be perfect or that I'm not and never will be?"

Similar to how negative, critical thoughts serve no purpose for your well-being and are counter-productive to creating what you want in your life, judgmental thoughts are equally unproductive and can create a rigidity or strictness in your thinking, and an unwillingness to see that which is good in yourself or another person. This type of thinking is also small-minded, and not expansive in developing your consciousness in any way. If you judge yourself or others, explore your reasons why. Are your judgments based on what is real and actual, or influenced by your beliefs, which might be fixed or narrow and need to be looked at more closely so that you can be more open-minded, and perhaps even forgiving of yourself or of others who might be different than you? Investigate your thoughts always, especially those that are most charged or heated with judgment, and by questioning them with the *Says Who?* method you can find out if your judgmental thought:

*Is yours.*
*Someone else's.*
*Is a thought you like.*
*Is working for you.*
*Controls you.*
*You want to keep it or let go.*

**You** decide.

# Chapter 7

# The "Something to Worry About" Thoughts

*It only seems as if you're doing something when you're worrying.*
**—Lucy Maud Montgomery**

When we wake up each day, our thoughts mostly concern the quotidian tasks, such as things we have to do or how we're going to spend the day. Depending on what your very first activity is when you wake up, your focus is usually on what's in front of you. Things like making a cup of coffee, waking the kids up for school, going outside to get the paper, or walking the dog are the kinds of morning activities we're usually busy with when we first get up.

However, sometimes if we've gone to sleep with a thought in our mind that has us worried or concerned, it can be that very same thought that's with us when we wake. So even while we're performing our daily morning rituals, that worried thought can be percolating in our mind like the cup of coffee we're making. If that thought is something genuinely to be concerned or worried about, like you or someone you love has a health problem and are going to have some medical tests done that day, or you fear that you might get fired from your job because you have problems with your boss, or that, according to the prophet Nostradamus, today is the day that the world could come to an end, then it's understandable how the foremost thought in your head is one of worry or concern (even though the Nostradamus prediction is based more on prophecy than the reality of what is in the present, like a health or work problem). Whether your worry is based in reality or prophecy, what still remains is that you need to find out if the worrying thought you're having is really worth all the energy you're expending.

Yet, sometimes the thoughts bothering us are not based on anything concrete, like health or career problems. But they're in our mind anyway, even when we're making our breakfast or doing the Sunday crossword puzzle, and it's unsettling us enough to make us feel agitated or irritated, and maybe even angered by it. It just won't go away. I call those thoughts the "Something to Worry About" thoughts. They are those thoughts that give us something to worry or be concerned about because we feel we need to. If we're used to having something to worry about because it gives us a feeling that we're solving some kind of a problem—when, in fact, all we're doing is worrying needlessly—then we will find something to worry about.

It's not that worrying can't be useful, like using it as a motivator for studying for a test so that you'll do well on it, or getting something done by a deadline, but there are more productive ways to do well at something, or getting something done on time other than worrying or creating needless anxiety. Unless you consider yourself a genuine "worrier," which would be someone who's always anticipating something bad that *could* happen in the future, then you need to ask yourself if you're just someone who needs something to worry about because it's become more of a habit than anything else.

It's important to know the purpose and intention of your thoughts. If worrying is something you consciously want to spend your time doing, or you feel that it serves some kind of useful purpose for you, you will find that when you question thoughts that are based on worrying, how much time you actually spend and waste feeling anxious and concerned over things that you have absolutely no control over (like a natural disaster or an end of the world prediction), or that it has nothing to do with being in the present moment of your life and enjoying the things that you are doing right now.

Asking yourself *Says Who?* when you have a thought that's overtaken your mind with worry, is in essence asking yourself, "Who said I should worry like this?" This will begin the questioning process to understand the seriousness of your worry, and if your thought is really worth spending so much of your time on.

Again, if it's something to be genuinely concerned about, your questioning of it will let you know that your thought is important to you, and your concern is worth thinking about. But if you ask yourself, "Am I in control of this thought?" you might find out that your worrying is controlling your thoughts, instead of *you* being in control of them. By asking "Does this thought work for me?" you realize that, no, it isn't working for you because it's not solving anything for the better. Then, when you follow that question with, "Do I want to keep this thought or let it go?" you realize that yes, you need to let it go.

Keeping "something to worry about thoughts" in your mind can sometimes interfere not only with the things that are good in your life in the present, but they can also interfere with, and get in the way of, closeness or intimacy you can have with other people. It can be a type of barrier you place between yourself and someone else by having your worry or anxiousness over something that is preoccupying or even obsessing you be the focus or the topic of conversation that replaces talking about something more meaningful or relevant. It's one thing to share a genuine concern with someone close to you, but if it becomes a constant worry—real or imagined—without a resolution, you need to ask yourself why that thought is there, and is taking up so much space in your mind. Again, unless it serves a useful purpose for you, it doesn't belong there.

### Banish the "Something to Worry About" Thoughts:

By answering these questions, you'll find out if you're ready to let go of those "Something to Worry About" thoughts. If they have no use for your well-being—they're just keeping you busy worrying.

1. Says who?
   *"Who said I should worry like this? Am I telling myself to worry?"*
2. Have I heard someone say this thought before?
   *"Have I heard or witnessed someone I know worry about a thought like this before or something similar?"*
3. Do I like this thought?
   *"Do I like having a worried thought like this in my mind?"*
4. Does this thought make me feel better?
   *"Does having this worried thought in my mind make me feel better or add value to my life in any way?"*
5. Does this thought work for me?
   *"Does thinking this worried thought work for me in a positive, useful or productive way?"*
6. Am I in control of this thought?
   *"Is this worried thought controlling me or am I in control of it?"*
7. Do I want to keep thinking this thought, or let it go?
   *"Do I want to keep worrying about this, or do I want to release it and let it go?"*

The question "Have I heard someone say this thought before?" might shed some light on connecting your worried thought to someone you know, like a parent, grandparent or a family member, who was a worrier. Perhaps you grew up seeing them in that state a lot, and just assumed it was normal. Now you realize this habit of worrying has become yours. Find out what good your worrying is doing for you by questioning it. You may discover that it's doing absolutely nothing good or productive for you—it's just keeping you in a worried state, and by reducing worry, it will minimize anxiety and stress in your life. I've seen this happen with many of my clients.

I had a client who was a constant worrier. She told me that she had always been that way, even when she was a young girl, but really wanted to learn how to minimize worrying so much because it made her feel stressed all the time. When I asked her the *Says Who?* questions, one by one, she was able to answer each of them almost immediately, which clearly indicated to me that she was more than ready to do something about her worrying. Her answers revealed:

*Says who?*—That she was completely aware that she was saying her worried thoughts in her mind, therefore taking full responsibility for having them.

*Have I heard someone say this thought before?*—That she had grown up with a parent that was a constant worrier, and had been influenced by them.

*Do I like this thought?*—That she never liked her worried thoughts, and actually loathed having them.

*Does this thought make me feel better?*—That she was completely aware that her worried thoughts not only didn't make her feel better, they made her feel anxious constantly.

*Does this thought work for me?*—That she knew that her worried thoughts did not work for her in a positive, productive way, and felt that they were hurting her, even at times making her feel sick to her stomach.

*Am I in control of this thought?*—That she felt so taken over by her worried thoughts most of the time that she didn't believe she could stop them from having a hold on her.

*Do I want to keep this thought or let it go?*—That she felt desperate to be able to let go of her worried thoughts.

My client was genuinely ready to stop worrying so much, and was willing to do whatever it took to make that happen, but what was most revealing about what she "believed" about her worried thoughts was that she didn't know what it would feel like if she actually stopped worrying, which made her feel anxious—causing her to *worry about no longer worrying!* I had her work the *Says Who?* method on that thought too, and she eventually came to understand how she kept perpetuating her worrying, even when she thought she wasn't. She kept working the method when any of her thoughts even slightly conjured up worry for her, and she soon saw how they started to diminish. This gave her tremendous relief, and gave her an empowered feeling of being in control of her "Something to worry about" thoughts for the first time in her life.

If you're really sick and tired of worrying, you can stop yourself from doing it once you realize you don't want to do it anymore, and if you genuinely have something that deserves your concern, give it the time you need to work it through in your mind, and then let it go. By that I mean: don't spend more time on it then need be. Know the difference between worrying needlessly, and caring about something you hope will be okay, which can be the thought you hold in your mind. Try and replace your worried thought with thoughts of love and healing, which are more productive thoughts than thoughts of worrying.

This is especially true when we are consumed with worry over a loved one's health. Instead of wasting energy on worry, a much more useful and effective way to use our mind can be to hold healing thoughts about an ill loved one instead of anxious ones. It feels like you're actually doing something to help them when you hold healing thoughts for them, rather than thoughts of worry, which are thoughts you can't really shape or construct into anything other than perpetuating a feeling of helplessness. That can also give you more anxiety. Holding healing thoughts makes you feel that you're doing something positive and proactive to help the person who needs it. And if you find yourself worrying about your own well-being with a health situation or crisis, try and take some quiet time to apply the same healing thoughts for yourself.

Here are some ways to turn your "Something to Worry About Thoughts" into healing thoughts:

1. When you have a worried thought about someone (or yourself) acknowledge it by saying, "I am worried about (say name)."
2. Tell yourself, "I surround (say name) in white light and love and see them healing."
3. Tell yourself, "I hold (say name) in my mind as a vibrant, healthy person."
4. Tell yourself, "(Say name) has my love and blessings."

Try and do this when you find yourself worrying about someone or yourself. It will help you focus on their or your wellness instead of worrying needlessly. It's also helpful to do before you go to bed so that your worried thought doesn't keep you up and anxious, unable to fall asleep.

And remember, when a worried thought pops up in your mind, try to first **Acknowledge it**, **Observe it,** and not **React to it**. This will help you stay present and neutral with your worry so it won't plug you into it even more, making it seem bigger than it probably is. By remaining calm, even if you're dealing with something that has reason for concern or worry, you will be able to handle it better, and with a much clearer mind.

## PART II

# Acknowledge
# Your Thoughts

*The ancestor of every action is a thought.*
**—Ralph Waldo Emerson**

## Chapter 8
# Owning Your Thoughts

*Attack the evil that is within yourself,*
*rather than attacking the evil that is in others."*
**—Confucius**

Our thoughts create our "reality" in our minds, and whether we like it or not, we're stuck with those thoughts unless we want to do something about changing them. What we know is that if you don't like some of your thoughts, you can change them by questioning them with the *Says Who?* method and decide if you want to keep them or let them go. But in order for you to begin that process, you have to first **Own Your Thoughts.**

What that means is that until you **acknowledge** the thoughts you have, you don't really have control over them—they basically *own you.* Owning your thoughts is admitting to yourself that you're willing to take a good close look at all of them and decide if you're being honest about them. Thinking certain thoughts, and then living your life differently than how you think, or distancing yourself from your thoughts—which can best be described as "Not walking your talk," or better yet, "Not walking your thoughts,"—is living your life dishonestly or hypocritically, especially if what you think or say is not what you do or how you behave.

*If your actions don't reflect your thoughts,*
*then there's a disconnect between them.*

Some people live their lives split between what they think and how they act, and might not even know that there's a schism or a contradiction between their thoughts and actions because they're not honest about their thoughts—other than what they tell you or would like you, or even themselves, to believe about them. When I'm in the presence of someone who doesn't seem like they've done much self reflection about their thoughts or examined their conflicted or confused thinking, what that tells me is that they're not connecting to themselves as honestly as they could be, not necessarily because they don't want to, but that they might not know "how" to.

Connecting to yourself means connecting to your thoughts, and by connecting to them, you know what they really are. Only then can you truly **own** them as yours. If you don't want to own them, then that means you're not really satisfied or happy with them, and if that's the case, wouldn't you rather change them for the better than deny having them? Well, the truth is you really can't begin to change your thoughts for the better unless you own them, and once you do, you can start the process of questioning them with the *Says Who?* method, and then decide if you want to **keep them** or **let them go**.

That means stripping away any dishonesty you may have about yourself and finding out if you've been avoiding the truth of who you are. *In other words: How honest are you with yourself and the thoughts you have—all of them?*

If you don't own your negative thoughts, then you're denying having them—which doesn't mean they're going to go away. Quite the opposite, actually. They might stay pushed down, or dormant for a while, but eventually they will rear their negative head, and sometimes with more force than you would like, and yet, some people will choose to keep pushing them down or away because it's the easier or more convenient thing to do.

But you can't change anything about yourself for the better if you're not being honest about the thoughts you have, good *and* bad. If you feel that avoiding or denying your negative thoughts works for you, then I can only assume that on some level you've just gotten used to thinking either negative, critical, judgmental or even mean-spirited thoughts and accepted them as a normal way of thinking, even though they may be unhealthy, or even detrimental to your well-being. *But, remember: just because you're used to those thoughts does not mean you have to continue accepting them!* You can change them at any time, but first you have to be willing to claim them as yours.

Can you recall when you were a child in elementary school, and a student blurted out something inappropriate in the classroom, and when the teacher turned around and said "Who said that!?" nobody wanted to admit it was them because they didn't want to get into trouble? Well, now's the time to come clean with yourself because you're not going to get into trouble—you're actually doing something good for yourself.

Everyone has thoughts that pop up in their mind, and as we know, they're not always kind or nice, but by owning those types of thoughts, you're admitting to yourself that your mind stores certain thoughts or ideas you might not be happy or proud of, or maybe even embarrassed to admit. Perhaps you are more comfortable keeping those thoughts to yourself. But, whether you prefer keeping your thoughts private or sharing them with someone, the most important person you need to come clean with is yourself. That means you own your thoughts—all of them, including the ones you might not want to admit having. This isn't about hiding some thoughts and coming clean about others. This is about revealing all of them to yourself. Just like cleaning out that closet or basement (your subconscious storage room), you've got to really get in there, establish order, and take everything out that is not serving your purpose before you can begin to put anything back that will ultimately be useful to your well-being.

The danger of not owning your negative thoughts is that not doing it will keep them shrouded in shame or embarrassment; that's the "hidden" aspect that ends up making them seem worse than they really are. Another reason they make you feel bad is because you've probably labeled or judged them (and yourself) harshly without exploring what they're really about by questioning them.

For some, that can mean thoughts of jealousy, competition, judgment, greed or even hate. Just having those types of thoughts is so uncomfortable for some people, they'd just as soon push those thoughts away and pretend they aren't theirs. Those thoughts are considered common and normal (everyone at one point or another in their lives has had those kinds of thoughts or feelings), but the difference between thinking them and owning them is how you handle them. In other words, do you just let certain negative or unkind thoughts slip in and out of your mind without feeling bad or uncomfortable about them? Or, do you catch yourself having those kinds of thoughts and recognize that it's beneath you to think that way, aware that thinking those kinds of thoughts doesn't really make you feel good about yourself? If so, that's owning it.

*Acknowledging your negative, critical, petty, or*
*mean-spirited thoughts is having an awareness of them.*

That helps you to be honest about them, which is the first step to change them if you want to. But separating yourself from those negative or critical types of thoughts, or even denying them to yourself, as if you're really not thinking them (when in fact you are), is dishonest, and definitely not owning them.

So how do you Own Your Thoughts, including the ones you'd prefer pretending you don't have? You hold the thought in your mind, as uncomfortable as it may be, and ask yourself "Says who?" which is saying "Who is saying this (insensitive, critical, or nasty) thought in my mind?" then answer honestly to yourself, "I am," which is admitting that it's your thought, and you're willing to take a really close look at it, which is taking responsibility for having it. It's like saying, "Yes, that's me thinking this (insensitive, critical, or nasty) thought," and maybe even going further with your honesty and saying "It's not so nice, I know."

Say you're thinking something critical or mean, like, "She's so skinny; I hate her," or "They're so happily married, I can't stand them," or "He has so much success, I hope he fails." By using the *Says Who?* method when you find yourself having these negative, petty or mean-spirited thoughts, you are coming face-to-face with the realization that it is *you* that is holding this thought, and therefore forced to own it as yours, as unappealing or unkind as it may be. You can then ask yourself "Do I like this thought?" which will help you realize that thinking negative, petty or mean-spirited thoughts isn't positive or kind, and what's so likable about that? Asking yourself "Does this thought work for me?" might help you realize that it really doesn't work in your favor to think thoughts that are petty, jealous, greedy or mean-spirited, and that you need to make a change.

I once had a client who was very critical of himself, and sometimes when he'd share his thoughts with me he would preface it by saying how "bad" or "wrong" and even "dark" some of them were. He had already labeled and judged his thoughts before he even told me what they were. His judgment about having them was far more negative and degrading than the very thought itself. He decided that he was a "bad" person for having negative thoughts, so not only was he judgmental about his thoughts, but he was even harder on himself for having them. That's like adding insult to injury, which only made him feel worse about himself. Owning your thoughts is **not** about beating yourself up afterwards. It's about admitting to yourself that you have certain thoughts you aren't necessarily proud of, and then making efforts to change them. Just like there are people who don't own their thoughts because they'd prefer to separate themselves from having them, there are also people who own them with tremendous judgment, and if that's the case for you, it's important to not only own your negative thought, but to also own that you're being judgmental about them, which is really being honest with yourself!

If each of us tended to our own minds to make sure we were thinking positive, compassionate, kind, and life-affirming thoughts, I have no doubt the world would be a better place. Unfortunately, that isn't the case. Yes, there are people who are very mindful and committed to raising the consciousness on the planet by taking responsibility for how they think, their actions, and how they live their lives. They realize that the only way to make a positive difference is to do what Gandhi advised: "Be the change you want to see in the world." But what that really means is that change starts with each of us by changing our thoughts for the better.

If you don't question your thoughts, then you're accepting them as real and true, but if they aren't based in reality, and are a distorted perception of how you see the world or how you think things should be done, then you can not only affect your own well-being, but also disrupt the peace and well-being of others, and can even create serious problems, especially if you're in a position of authority or power like a parent, boss, or political leader.

That's why going to a therapist or having someone you can confide in to talk about what you're really thinking and feeling, as unpleasant or uncomfortable as it may be, can be helpful for getting those types of thoughts and feelings out so they're not pent up or imprisoned in your mind.

Having to keep your unpleasant or uncomfortable thoughts bottled up or hidden means that you're walking around burdened with secrets about yourself. The problem is that you can then start to be critical and judgmental of those very thoughts you're trying to hide, which only makes the situation worse, and can make you think that your secrets are bad or dark, when, in fact, maybe they're not as bad or dark as you think they are, which was the case for my client who thought his were, and would berate himself because of it. Or, even if they are, examining them in the light of day can help you deal with them. If you can't own those types of thoughts, and recognize them as negative and unhealthy, then you run the risk of them becoming very real for you to the point where they can control most of your thinking and influence your reality, which can be destructive and dangerous—not only to yourself, but to others.

But not everyone can go to a therapist, or has a confidant they feel comfortable to tell some of their deep, dark thoughts to. You certainly can start by being your own confidant by owning your thoughts instead of denying them or pushing them away, which is such an important step to take in learning how to process your thoughts and how to manage them. That's why going through the steps of letting those thoughts go begins with the number one essential thing: **Owning Your Thoughts**.

By taking an honest, close look at them, you can begin the process of questioning them, which is the only way to discover:

1. What they're doing in your mind.
2. If they're real or not.
3. If they're serving your well-being.

Owning your thoughts is being honest and truthful with yourself. At the end of the day, you're the one that has to look yourself in the mirror, and sleep comfortably at night. I think the reason why most people act out their destructive thoughts is because they think they can get away with doing whatever they want to do, as crazy or delusional as their idea might be. This is another indication how your mind can play tricks on you when you least expect it. That is why it is so important to know your mind, and all of the many thoughts that come in and out of it daily. Some of them want nothing more than to lead you astray, and if you're not careful in catching them, **owning** them, and questioning them, they can take you down a destructive road you may end up wishing you never traveled. Remember, you're in the driver's seat of your mind, and the mind is a powerful thing to control. Own your thoughts or they will own your mind.

## Mental Clean-Up:
## Taking Responsibility for your Thoughts

We shower, brush our teeth, clean our home, wash our cars and pets, and yet, when it comes to cleaning out the negative thoughts that occupy our mind, some people would rather sweep them under the proverbial rug than go anywhere near their mental messes, which is why they avoid owning their thoughts for as long as they possibly can. The problem with avoiding getting your thoughts in order, just like you would your home, is that all sorts of negative clutter or chaos starts to happen rather quickly. Even though your mind doesn't get filthy the way a house can with dust and dirt, it certainly can get sloppy and disorganized, and yes, "dirty" in its own way to the point that you can feel overwhelmed or unable to handle or manage your negative, confused or distorted thoughts properly, and need help to clear out your mind. But not everyone thinks they need the help they do, and they walk around a mental mess without even realizing it. Unfortunately, that affects not only themselves negatively, but everyone around them.

Mental negligence is highly irresponsible, because the mind is a powerful thing, which, if not tended properly, not only can wreak havoc on you and your life, it can also disrupt other people's lives and well-being too. To think that your negative thoughts don't affect others is naïve. All we have to do is take a look at how some of the most powerful leaders and dictators of the world have run their countries and people into the ground with poverty, violence and genocide, and we can see how the thoughts of just one person can affect the lives of millions of people, and the outcome can be catastrophic and tragic.

We'd like to believe that people who are in power, whether they're running a country, business, family or even a pilot of an airplane with hundreds of people on board in their care, have clear, healthy minds working, and are consciously aware that how they think and the decisions they make must be laser sharp.

People from Genghis Khan to Hitler to Osama Bin Laden have endangered, murdered and annihilated millions of people due to their distorted, perverse, even downright evil thinking. What we have to remember is that even the most heinous of crimes started with **someone having a single thought** run amuck in their mind, and took hold with such fierce, unquestioned intensity that not only did they believe their thought as real and righteous, but they were able to convince others (often millions of others) that their insane reality was just.

Questioning our thoughts with *Says Who?* not only protects our own well-being, it also serves as a "reality check". Each of us needs to know our own minds so that we can recognize what is true or distorted in another person. If we can't identify the difference in ourselves, how can we see it in someone else?

Remember: If we don't question our own thoughts to find out if they're real or not, and have a reality check by challenging our thoughts from time to time, then how can we recognize someone else's distorted thinking or reality? And if we can't identify the difference between real and unreal thoughts in ourselves, we definitely won't be able to recognize them in someone else, which is why listening to, emulating, or following anyone whose thoughts are negative or distorted can be unwise and potentially dangerous.

It all starts with us. Know your thoughts, and that means all of them. Especially the ones that try to commandeer your thinking, and tell you who you are, which is less than what you would prefer thinking about yourself. The minute a thought pops up in your mind that tells you that you're bad or not good enough, know right then and there that those types of thoughts need to be confronted and challenged immediately so that they don't distort your perception of who you really are.

Having a skewed perception of ourselves can alter how we see others, and the world in general. It can influence our whole ability to judge properly, and that can mean from a moral or ethical standpoint. What's deeply concerning about that is if we no longer are able to discern what is real and what is not, we can then lose our ability to determine what is right or wrong, and what can follow that is ultimately not being able to know clearly what is sane or insane.

A sane world requires having a sane consciousness collectively. But, in order for that to happen, each of us has to take responsibility for doing our own **Mental Clean-Up**—that is, a "reality check", which means cleaning up and clearing out any negative or distorted thoughts that need to be questioned and challenged with the *Says Who?* method so that we can know what is real and what is not. We must be fully "awake" to our own thoughts, and that means being completely conscious of them—in other words, literally being "on to" them, which requires being as honest about them as we possibly can. By questioning them, we see them for what they "really" are, and what purpose they're serving in our mind—"constructive or destructive."

We must know our thoughts, and the intentions behind them, which we only can by questioning them, and that is why the *Says Who?* method is so helpful and effective. Not knowing yourself fully means that you lived an "unexamined life," and chose not to probe or look further into the thoughts you hold in your mind, especially the ones that are negative.

Here are some thoughts you may have had and not want to "own." See if any of them have crossed your mind. Be honest!

1.  I'm better than you.
2.  I'm jealous of you.
3.  I don't like you.
4.  I don't like myself.
5.  I hate you.
6.  I hate myself.
7.  I hate minorities.
8.  I hate gay people.
9.  I resent you.
10. I resent myself.
11. I hope you fail.
12. I hope I fail.
13. I don't want you to be successful.
14. I don't want to be successful.
15. I want what you have: life, job, house, car, husband, wife, boyfriend, girlfriend, children, etc.
16. I wish you weren't here.
17. I wish I wasn't with you.
18. I wish I didn't know you.
19. I wish I never met you.
20. I wish I wasn't married to you.
21. I wish I wasn't in a relationship with you.
22. I wish I wasn't related to you.
23. I wish you would move to another country.
24. I wish you were never born.
25. I wish I were never born.
26. I want to dominate you.
27. I want you to dominate me.
28. I want to hurt you.

29. I want you to hurt me.
30. I want to hurt myself.
31. I want you to need me.
32. I don't want to need you.
33. I wish you were dead.
34. I wish I were dead.
35. I wish they (person, minority, group, etc.) didn't exist.
36. I fear you.
37. I fear myself.
38. I want to do something dangerous.
39. I want to break the law.
40. I want to do something crazy.
41. I want to rule the world.
42. I want to destroy the world.
43. I want to destroy you.
44. I want to destroy myself.

There are many other thoughts like these you can add to this list that you might not want to "own," and maybe I didn't mention some that you may have had. Again, having an unkind, mean, nasty, or even destructive thought doesn't mean you're a bad or evil person, but it does mean that you need to take a close look at your negative thoughts, and find out why you have them, and then decide by questioning them with the *Says Who?* method what you want to do with them—keep them, or let them go. Holding onto negative thoughts creates negative energy, and even if you deny having them, sometimes people can pick up on your energy, which can be negative because of the thoughts you're holding in your mind. If you asked yourself "Says who?" and attached any of the thoughts on this list to them, it would be interesting to see what comes up for you when you say to yourself, "I am having this thought." It might help you realize how toxic your thought is, and that you don't want to hold onto it anymore. That can feel very liberating.

**Own your thoughts.** They belong to no one but you so you may as well get to know what they're about because *what they are, is who you are* and don't you want to find out what that is? Be brave—go towards your thoughts to see them for what they really are. There is no teacher to get you in trouble. You are the teacher now—of your mind!

And remember: Each of us is our own leader, and must guide ourselves towards a healthy, productive life worth living, and that requires that our mind function clearly with thoughts that are positive, healthy and life-affirming. We cannot rely on others to define what is real for us. If we do, we might find ourselves being influenced or led by someone with a distorted perception of reality, nor should we lead someone with our own distorted perceptions. Ultimately, we all need to "own" our thoughts by doing our "mental clean up" and define what is real for us by questioning our thoughts, and the *Says Who?* method will always help do that.

## Chapter 9
# Thoughts vs. Feelings

*I don't want to be at the mercy of my emotions.*
*I want to use them, to enjoy them, and to dominate them.*
**—Oscar Wilde**

O ur thoughts affect our emotions because whatever we tell ourselves we believe, and, depending on what we believe, that influences how we feel.

But sometimes our feelings seem like they're controlling us because what we're feeling is so intense and emotional, we assume that our feelings have the upper hand, which, in fact, they do, because when we are functioning out of pure emotion our thinking function literally seems to fade when our emotions have taken over. When we're feeling happy and joyous, it's usually easy to link those feelings to particular thoughts like, "I'm in love, It's a beautiful day, I'm going on vacation, I got a raise," etc., but, when we're feeling something like sadness, sometimes it's not as easy to get to the exact reason for our unhappiness because we can feel so weighed down or overwhelmed by it, that all you can register is how stuck you feel in your misery. It's like being in quicksand and feeling that you're slipping deeper and deeper into a hole without even really knowing how you got there or how you're going to get out.

Feeling an emotion like sadness, to the point where it's taken over your mood and you can't seem to shake it off, is often not just because of the very thing that made you sad, like the end of a relationship, or the death of a loved one, etc., but it can be the ongoing thoughts around what caused your sadness that can linger or dominate your mind. It's those thoughts connected to your emotion that you need to question or even challenge with the *Says Who?* method so you can process it properly because it's very easy to get sucked into, or even taken over by an emotion like sadness, to the point where it can escalate into something more serious like depression, if you're not careful.

The end of anything meaningful, or loss of someone that was deeply important to us, can conjure up so many thoughts related to it that are purely emotion driven. For example: The death of a loved one can be so profoundly devastating for us, that a thought like, "I don't want to be here anymore if they're not here," can get planted in our mind almost immediately when someone close to us dies, and that thought will remain attached to our emotion, even if it's buried inside our heart. That's why for some people, they cannot get over their sadness or grieving over the loss of a loved one, so much so that they can go years still feeling deep sadness, not just because of losing someone they love, but because of their "thought" related to their loss, which is that they too want to die. Until you work through a thought as serious as that by examining it, you will continue to be at the effect of it.

Here's how you can use the *Says Who?* questions to challenge the thought, "I don't want to be here anymore if they're not here":

**Says who?** - Who is telling me that I don't want to be here anymore, if they're not here?

*Answer*: I am saying that I don't want to be here anymore if they're not here.

**Have I heard someone say this before?**

*Answer:* Yes, the person I lost said that to me. We loved each other so much that we didn't want to live without one another.

**Do I like this thought?**

*Answer:* No, I don't like the thought that I don't want to be here anymore if they're not here, even though that's how I feel without them.

**Does this thought make me feel better?**

*Answer:* Thinking that I don't want to be here anymore if they're not here doesn't make me feel better. It makes me feel very sad and even scared.

**Does this thought work for me?**

*Answer:* Thinking that I don't want to be here anymore if they're not here makes me feel horrible and so down. How can this thought possibly be working for me?

**Am I in control of this thought?**

*Answer:* Thinking that I don't want to be here anymore if they're not here is something I have felt for a long time. It's a very powerful thought for me. I don't think I'm in control of it.

**Do I want to keep this thought or let it go?**

*Answer:* I really don't want to keep thinking that I don't want to be here anymore if they're not here. I miss them so much, but I don't think I have to keep thinking this heavy thought all the time. What good is it? I want to let it go.

You can see how the *Says Who?* questions can be very helpful for processing a thought as serious as "I don't want to be here anymore if they're not here." And by going through each question, you can come to the realization that it's okay, and even time for you to let your thought go.

But sometimes people can't easily connect their emotion to something specific, and if you ask them what thought is associated to their feeling of sadness or whatever they're feeling, they might say something like "I don't know, I just feel sad," or "I feel anxious," or "I feel scared," which means they can tell you *what* they're feeling, but not always the reason *why* they're feeling what they are.

The reason they will tell you what they "feel" when asked is because their emotion is what feels so real for them in the moment. It's only when you ask them, "*Why* are you feeling sad or anxious or scared," that they might be able to step outside of their emotion and connect their feeling to a particular thought like "I feel sad because my child is going off to college and I'll miss seeing them every day, and having them close to me," or "I feel scared because I don't think I'm strong enough to stop drinking," or "I feel anxious because I don't think I'm ever going to find another job," etc.

When thoughts like that aren't questioned and challenged with the *Says Who?* method right away (and when the emotion related to those thoughts start to kick in), what you can then experience is emotion taking you over, and now you are at the mercy of your emotions because they're dominating you. That's why it's important to know when you're feeling something without understanding the thought or reason behind it, and take yourself through the steps needed to find out what the thought or thoughts are connected to your emotions, like sadness or anger, so your emotions don't escalate further. What you need to do when you are deep in your emotional state is:

1. Acknowledge what you're feeling.
2. Observe what you're feeling.
3. Don't react to what you're feeling.

By doing this, you're allowing yourself to be with, or "hold" the emotion you're having with an awareness of it, and that can help you get to the thought connected to it so you can question it with the *Says Who?* method, and find out if your thought is real or not, or someone else's thought you're holding onto, and if you're ready to let it go.

This process helps you stay calm so that you can see things more clearly, and will also help you understand that the thought you have around your emotion, which might feel very real for you, might not allow for another more positive, productive thought to help what you're feeling. For example, a thought like: "I'm sad because my child is going off to college and I won't see them every day, and will miss having them close to me," can be followed by a thought you can tell yourself like: "I know it will be hard at first, but with time it will get easier for both of us." This is a thought that can actually help an emotion like sadness so that it doesn't weigh on you heavily, last longer than need be, or even go into depression.

The *Says Who?* method helps you have a type of dialogue with yourself where you can be your own problem solver. You might have the very answer you need to help you with the emotion you're experiencing that's causing you unhappiness or distress, and by questioning it, you can allow for the types of positive thoughts that might not be in the foreground of your mind to come up and actually "advise" you what to do, like the thought, "I know it will be hard at first, but with time it will get easier for both of us."

There is so much **"gold"** for you to mine in your many thoughts, and you have way more positive, productive ones in your mind you're not using or might not even know about, especially when you're at the effect of an emotion that you're gripped by like sadness. Let the *Says Who?* method help you find your gold. It's there to be found!

Another way to know that there's something going on for you on an emotional level is how you feel it in your body. For example, when you're anxious or frightened, your heart can beat fast, or you might even feel palpitations. Or, when you are sad, you can feel lethargic and unmotivated, and might just want to stay in bed, and not be around anyone. It might not register for you that the reason you're feeling this way is because there are thoughts deeper within you that you're not aware of that are the source of your unhappiness, but you can't quite get to it yet. That's when an emotion is almost speaking for you. It's letting you know in your body what's going on inside you. If you can connect that emotion to the thought that triggered it or is behind it, it can help you get to the reason for your unhappiness, as painful as it may be.

The problem with keeping a thought stuck on an emotional level is that it can stay stuck there for a long time, and until you can hear the thoughts that are making you sad, your heart can remain heavy because you're not having a dialogue with it. It's good (and healthy) for us to be able to talk to ourselves, especially when we're feeling bad—as difficult as that may seem to do when we're so at the affect of our emotions.

If you can try to ask yourself the *Says Who?* questions when you're feeling sad, you're showing yourself that you care enough to find out why you're feeling unhappy. By continuing the questioning process you can begin to **connect your thoughts to your emotions**. In doing so, you will start to see how your particular thoughts can have such a deep effect on how you feel about yourself. It might make you more emotional at first, and maybe make you cry (there's nothing wrong with a good cry once in a while, is there?), but you need to face the thought behind your tears. If you really listen to it, it will tell you what is making you sad, and help you release your sadness so that you can work through it and understand it better.

Here's how you can use the *Says Who?* questions to help you get to the thought(s) you don't know yet. When you try this on your own, take your time with the questions, and don't feel rushed to answer them.

Sometimes just by slowly presenting yourself with each question, the thought(s) behind your feeling can suddenly come up.

**Says who?**

*Answer*: Is there a thought in my mind that's connected to my feelings? I can't think of one particular thought right this minute, but I feel unhappy and a little nervous.

**Have I heard someone say this thought before?**

*Answer:* Am I holding someone else's thought that is making me feel unhappy or nervous? I don't think so. I think this unhappy and nervous feeling is because something is weighing heavily on me, but I'm not really sure exactly what it is.

**Do I like this thought?**

*Answer (and **Realization**)*: I don't really like thinking that I'm getting older...and I'm not sure how things are going to turn out...and if I'm going to feel secure financially...and if everything's going to be okay because it doesn't feel okay for me right now...and...**Oh my god! I think I just realized why I'm feeling unhappy, and nervous! It's all these thoughts swirling around in my mind!**

**Does this thought make me feel better?**

*Answer*: None of those thoughts make me feel better. I had no idea how much they were dominating my mind!

**Does this thought work for me?**

*Answer*: Those thoughts are making me unhappy and anxious. I don't think that's helping me at all.

**Am I in control of this thought?**

*Answer*: No, I'm not feeling in control of those thoughts, and now that I think of it, they've been on my mind a lot lately, but I didn't realize they were making me feel this unhappy and nervous.

**Do I want to keep this thought or let it go?**

*Answer:* I don't want to keep feeling unhappy and nervous about my future. I'd like to let those thoughts go, and trust that everything's going to work out fine.

You can see how just by asking yourself the *Says Who?* questions, even if you don't really know all of the thoughts behind your feelings, it can get you thinking in a kind of open, freefalling way, and the thought(s) connected to your feelings can suddenly come up. And, by knowing what those thoughts are, you can work through them to find out whether they are real or not, or blown out of proportion, and if they're serving your well being, which clearly they wouldn't be if your emotion is unhappiness or feeling nervous.

However, I'm not saying that you're not going to feel sadness, nervousness, anger or whatever emotion you might experience at certain times in your life because of an event or circumstance (like losing a loved one, a job loss, divorce, empty nest, illness, argument with loved one, etc.) that evokes those emotions. Experiencing these emotions is normal, and sometimes necessary.

**The *Says Who?* questions aren't meant to eradicate your feelings because feelings are essential and healthy to have.** They're meant to help you understand *why* you're having them, and can't stop being at the effect of your feelings, by knowing the thoughts evoking them. The key is to not let your emotions *overtake you* or *keep a hold on you* longer than they should or need to, and the only way you can make sure that doesn't happen is by questioning your thoughts that are continuing to trigger your emotions.

When we're functioning on pure emotions, our thinking can become fuzzy, confused, and agitated. That's why when your emotions take you over, arguing and fighting with someone in that state might not be productive and can get hurtful and ugly because you're emotions are fired up. People can say some terrible things to one another when their emotions are in control, and their thinking process has faded temporarily.

When your thoughts are clear, and you're not in an emotional or reactive state, you can get a lot more accomplished by talking something out with someone, and be more prone to listening to one another. This can be very difficult when you're emotional with anger, causing you to raise your voice or scream to make your point. Have you ever had an instance when you've been in an argument or tense conversation with someone and you can't seem to think of the right words to get your point across, but later, after the dust is settled, you think of the perfect rejoinder? That's because, in the heat of the moment, you're allowing emotion to take you over and you're not able to think clearly. That's your thoughts vs. feelings at work.

## Allowing Your Feelings to Override Your Thoughts

One of the most common areas where we don't listen to our thoughts, and much *prefer* letting our feelings to lead the way is when we're attracted to someone. When you're feeling a strong sexual pull to someone, even if you're thinking "What a jerk!" your feelings of desire or lust are so strong and dominate, that you might even wish that your thought would just "get lost" or "take a hike!" The problem with that is that yes, your thought can take a "hike" for maybe a little while, but once you've had a thought like "What a jerk!" it's almost impossible for it to "get lost." More often than not, that thought will come back to haunt you because you were right in thinking that, and your instincts were trying to tell you something.

I had a very attractive client who had a history of disappointing relationships because she told her thoughts to "get lost," one too many times, preferring to let her emotions lead the way. It was hard for her to be the **observer** of her feelings. When she came to me for coaching, she had never done that in any of her relationships. If she liked someone, or was attracted to them, she would let that be the motivation for what she would do next, and even if she had thoughts that came up to warn her that maybe the guy wasn't what he "appeared" to be, she would ignore those thoughts because she didn't think they were as important as her "feelings."

I worked with her on what it felt like to **observe** her feelings, and when she described her feelings of sexual desire, she said to me, "I want to act on this feeling. It's like an impulsive thing for me."

"Of course you do," I said, "and that's very natural, but you have thoughts sometimes that are connected to your feelings, and do you still want to act on them if your thought is negative or trying to warn you about someone?"

She looked at me like I was pushing her to be honest with herself, and that she needed to come clean.

"No, I don't," she said. "I don't want to act on a thought I have about a guy when it's negative, but my feelings of attraction are so strong and good, that that's what I want to act on."

"But that's what ends up disappointing you. You end up going back to the same thought you had about that person that you didn't want to listen to, and that's what ends your relationship."

"I've always let my emotions lead the way," she said, "but what's interesting for me is that I often have a bad or negative thought, like, this guy's trouble, or he's a manipulator, come up pretty quickly, but I choose to ignore it."

"That's great that you recognize your thoughts so quickly," I told her. "Some people can't even do that. Your thoughts are trying to tell you something very important for you to listen to. They're trying to take care of you." I taught her how to use the *Says Who?* questions, and when she asked herself "Says who?" she answered, "My inner voice is telling me to act on my sexual impulse. But, it's hurt me in the past, so why should I trust this voice inside my head that's telling me to ignore my helpful thoughts?"

The great outcome of her story is that she's been in a positive, well-rounded relationship for a year now. She became such a good **observer** of her feelings that she chose not to act on them quickly or be impulsive, even though she was attracted to him. Instead, she had him court her for a while before they became intimate. This way, she got to know him really well first, and when a thought came up that she needed to pay attention to, she told him what she was thinking, which he really liked and found refreshing! He respected her honesty, and was willing to work with her in making the relationship a good one for both of them.

When you realize that your thoughts and emotions work in conjunction with each other, just like your conscious and subconscious work together, you become more aware of how they affect one another. With that understanding, you recognize that you need to be in control of keeping a delicate "thought/emotion" balance in your life so that one isn't dominating the other, and throwing you off center. This can happen when your thoughts and emotions work together in a positive way, as opposed to experiencing turmoil because of thoughts that are not examined properly, and are affecting your emotions in a negative way. By knowing your thoughts, you can know and understand your emotions better. It's important to merge them together when they've lost their communication. The *Says Who?* method will help them have an active dialogue.

*Chapter 10*

# Stop Over Identifying With Your Negative Thoughts

*Make not your thoughts your Prisons.*
—**William Shakespeare**

Now that you understand how powerful, important and valuable your thoughts are, and how they affect your emotions and influence everything in your life, it's important that you always try to connect what you're feeling to a thought, if you can. And if you can't, ask yourself the *Says Who?* questions to begin your process of discovery.

When you get to the thought connected to your emotion, remember the first thing to do is:

1. Acknowledge it.
2. Be the Observer.
3. Not the Reactor.

If you are going through something that is challenging or are having a difficult time in your life, that is usually when your thoughts can be most active—teeming with worry, fear, doubt, anxiety or even confusion. It's very easy at those times for your mind to go on "automatic," and let your negative thoughts take you over. This can make being an observer extremely difficult. Those are the times when you have to be even that much more vigilant in resisting the temptation to believe every single negative or fear-based thought racing through your mind as true or real—especially if you're in reactive mode. It's those moments—especially when you are feeling like you're about to lose control because of something upsetting or challenging that's happening in your life—when the *Says Who?* method is essential. That's when you need to be even more in control of your thoughts, and stop them from getting you into a state of mind that can be not only fearful and diminishing, but could in fact be destructive, causing you to act impulsively because you feel so frustrated, frightened, or even hopeless.

> *Remember, when we are being challenged or having a hard time, that's when our thoughts stir up our emotions, and we begin to not only believe what we're thinking, but can mistake our feelings as real, when in fact, it's our emotions being directly affected by our thoughts of fear, worry, or doubt.*

Your emotions can get amplified and heated, and put you into a complete panic or chaotic state of mind that can take you over. Suddenly you feel out of control, like a hostage to your fired-up emotions moving through your body. It can get so bad that you begin to feel you're not going to ever be OK, causing your panic to escalate. If you've ever observed someone spinning out of control or acting like they're losing it and have tried to help them, you can see what an intense and frightened state of mind they're in, and how difficult it is to get through to them. Trying to "talk someone down" means that you're trying to appeal to the rational thinking part of their mind, which is clear, sane and lucid. But when someone is in reactive mode because their thoughts are firing away at them kamikaze-style, and they're believing they're real, it's pretty difficult to get their attention to focus on anything other than what they're reacting to and believing about their thoughts. That's when sticking them in a cold shower can seem like the only thing to do to get through to them.

Although that's an extreme example of how agitated someone can get when they're in a negative state of mind that has them reeling and reacting, it is nonetheless something that can happen. This is caused by two, often simultaneous, events:

1. Not questioning your thought(s) to find out if they are real or not;
2. Over-identifying with your negative thought(s) so much so that you absolutely believe them to be true.

In this state of mind, you are as far removed from being an observer and separating yourself from your thoughts as you possibly can, and this can escalate into something serious because you are in complete reactive mode. *That's why it's so important that the minute that first negative thought pops into your head, you* **Acknowledge** *that it's there,* **Observe** *without reacting, and begin your* **Says Who?** *questions right away.*

When certain upsetting events happen in our lives, causing us to feel insecure, doubtful, fearful, sad, angry, or out of control, that's when we are more prone to listen to our negative thoughts and believe them as true. It's usually when something unexpected happens, like losing a job, causing a financial crisis, the end of relationship or marriage, a death of a loved one, or any unexpected change occurring that we weren't anticipating or mentally prepared for, that throws us off balance or makes us feel broadsided. That's when we fall prey to over-identifying with our negative or fear-based thoughts. We feel uncertain, doubt ourselves, and often interpret what's happening to us as our responsibility or fault.

It's those types of situations that can make us feel that we can't handle what's happening to us, and we begin to over-identify with those thoughts. If something is upsetting, disturbing, heartbreaking or frightening we can feel so overtaken by our emotions, as I explained, which are directly affected by our thoughts, that we lose sight of what is real and what is not, causing us to believe that what's happening is threatening to our well-being. By **observing**, then **acknowledging** those thoughts, you can isolate and identify the exact ones that make you feel frightened or out of control, and then immediately question them with the *Says Who?* method.

Example: Thinking that you're never going to work again because you lost your job. You're allowing the feelings of shock and despair to overwhelm your thoughts; you are over-identifying with what has happened to you, and believe that thought—that because you lost your job you will never get another one—as true. In other words, your whole sense of identity gets caught up and influenced by something negative that's happened to you, and you cannot separate yourself from it to see this is temporary and that there's probably a solution to your problem.

If you can stop yourself from reacting to your negative situation and allow yourself to challenge and question a thought like: "I will never work again," with the *Says Who?* method, you will find out that your thought is merely a reaction you're having to an incident that's happened, and it's distorted your perception of yourself. You can change this by questioning your thoughts.

| How to question the thought "I will never work again." | |
|---|---|
| **Question** | **Which Means** |
| Says who? | Who is telling me that I will never work again because I lost my job? Is it me telling myself that, and if so, why do I have to believe it's true? |
| Have I heard someone say this thought before? | Have I heard someone say that if I lose my job I will never work again, and if I have, why did I take their thought or belief on as my own? |
| Do I like this thought? | Do I like thinking that I'll never work again because I lost my job, and if I don't, why am I thinking it? |
| Does this thought make me feel better? | Does thinking that I will never work again because I lost my job make me feel better about myself, and if it doesn't, why am I thinking it? |
| Does this thought work for me? | Does thinking that I will never work again because I lost my job work for me in a positive or productive way, and if not, why am I thinking it? |

| Am I in control of this thought? | Does thinking that I will never work again because I lost my job control my thoughts, or am I in control of this thought, and if not, why am I letting a negative thought like this control my thinking? |
|---|---|
| Do I want to keep this thought or let it go? | Do I want to keep thinking that I will never work again because I lost my job, or do I want to let this thought go? |

The only way you can get over-identified with a negative thought, and let it define your sense of "self," is if you believe it as true and real. Questioning and challenging a negative thought with the *Says Who?* method helps you see clearly that your negative thoughts do not determine who you are, nor define your true identity. *You* define your authentic self, and your thoughts should support who you truly are, in spite of a temporary setback or unexpected crisis. Even if an isolated incident happens that shakes you up, causing you to be fearful or to doubt yourself, it's the positive thoughts you tell yourself to counter the distorted perception you have of yourself (because of a negative incident) that will help you realize that you are in control of your mind always, and your thoughts create your reality. And even if your reality right now isn't ideal, or what you want it to be, you can't change it if your thinking is in reactive mode, reeling from something that's happened to you that you're not liking or are unhappy about. You need to keep your thoughts clear, positive and productive so you can create a solution and game plan for yourself to change your current situation for the better, which a positive, non-reactive thinking mind will help you do.

Question your negative thoughts before you convince yourself they're real and permanent. If they're not serving your well-being, they're not the type of thoughts you should allow to define you, and certainly not to hold onto. Those are the type of thoughts you need to question and challenge immediately with the *Says Who?* method so that you don't over identify with them and believe them as real and true when they're absolutely not!

## Chapter 11

# The Danger of Believing
# Your Negative Thoughts

*If you realized how powerful your thoughts are,*
*you would never think a negative thought.*
**—Peace Pilgrim**

Just because some inner voice in your head tells you that you are unworthy, unlovable, a loser, or whatever mean "sandbox name" it wants to call you, it doesn't mean that it's a fact or even based in reality. You have the power to challenge and change a negative thought always, as harsh or brutal as it may be.

As I've said, when there hasn't been a questioning process of your thoughts, and your emotions and behavior are a result of troubling or disturbing thoughts, it can become a negative state of mind that can dominate you. This can cause you to make impulsive, irrational, desperate, or even destructive and dangerous decisions because the only thing that is occupying your mind at a time of difficulty or despair is a thought that tells you things are not OK and are going to stay that way. This can lead to feeling unsafe, uncertain, or convinced that your survival is being threatened, even if that is not actually the case.

It's also important to note that the type of thoughts I'm referring to are the garden variety troubling thoughts that plague most of us. Each of us at times feels anxious, sad, worried, or frightened. Millions of people experience days when they don't want to get out of bed and just pull the covers over their head.

I want to make it clear that part of being alive and human is to feel all sorts of things at different times, depending on what's going on in your life, and that can even mean a gloomy day affecting your mood negatively. At different times we can alternately feel great, good, so-so, not so good, and even terrible. What I'm hoping with the *Says Who?* method is that it can be part of your daily practice, to be put to use *before* your negative thoughts can go so far as to push you into a more serious or troubled state of mind, causing you to opt for relief through medication, alcohol or any substance that can numb your feelings. Questioning your negative thoughts and dissolving them can change your state of mind for the better. It's certainly a good place to start before you decide to do something more extreme or radical like anesthetizing yourself with anything that is mind altering or numbing.

I'm not saying that people diagnosed with depression or a clinical type of mental illness can just change their thoughts right away and everything will be just fine. Maybe they can't, as they might have a chemical imbalance or some other medical condition. If that's the case, sometimes medication is absolutely necessary, especially if there is a more serious underlying problem like depression, or one is experiencing a feeling of ongoing, relentless hopelessness or despair. Hopefully, those with serious problems who need professional help are working with a mental health professional or someone qualified in this area to help. Yet, even with professional help, you can continue to think troubling thoughts on your own, away from any outside help you're receiving, and have no method or technique to question those thoughts, leaving you feeling overwhelmed or taken over by thoughts that make you feel bad, or so down that your life isn't worth living anymore.

Clearly, if you have reached a point in your life where your depression becomes serious, and perhaps destructive or suicidal thoughts have entered your mind, again, I can't emphasize enough how seeking professional help is extremely important, and should be sought immediately. Unfortunately, many people don't seek the help they need, and something that could have started as a bout of unhappiness or mild depression can often go unchecked or untreated, and thoughts that support their unhappiness or depression become too dominant in their thinking process. That person does not understand that "they are not their negative thoughts," meaning that they are too enmeshed and over-identified with them. There is no separation between the negative thought and a healthy sense of "self", which is who you are when you're not gripped by fear or despair. A negative thought is disruptive to feeling balanced, confident and whole, and can cause doubt and uncertainty. That can lead to situations where you might make unhealthy, destructive, or life threatening decisions because you do not know that "you are not your negative thoughts," and the separation between "thought" and "self" is blurred and unclear.

A thought like you're "bad, ugly, worthless, unlovable" or whatever critical or undermining thought you've told yourself or someone has said to you, must be confronted and challenged before it becomes fueled by more negative and critical thoughts, and they will definitely keep on coming if you don't tell them to stop. It's one thing to stand up for yourself if someone is attacking you and saying mean or hurtful things to you directly, but if you can't stand up to your own negative or critical thoughts, then you're allowing more harm to be done, and you will begin to believe what you're telling yourself. That's when you start to believe that "you are your negative thoughts," and accept them as real and true, which can not only be hurtful, but damaging to your self-esteem and self-worth. It's important to consider negative thoughts as a form of abuse. Just like you wouldn't tolerate anyone abusing someone you love, you have to ask yourself why you would allow for a type of mental abuse to be done to you—*by you*!

I had a client who was extremely hard on herself, and when things were not going so well for her, she felt like she was on a downward spiral "circling the drain," as she would describe it, and those were the times she would tell herself how absolutely "worthless" she was. I asked her to picture herself holding a child in her arms, and imagine someone coming along who tries to hurt that child, either verbally or physically.

"Wouldn't you immediately want to protect that child from being in harm's way," I asked her.

"Absolutely!" she said.

"Alright, then why wouldn't you want to protect yourself from abuse in the same way? Don't you think you need to protect yourself from being hurt just like you would protect someone you love?"

"Yes," she said, "but I guess I'm not very good at doing that. Obviously I need to love myself better."

Sometimes the demeaning and degrading things we tell ourselves can be far more scathing and hurtful than anything someone can say to us, but whatever type of verbal abuse we hear, whether it's coming from someone else, or from us to ourselves, it's always our choice and decision to decide if we want to take it in and believe it as true, or reject it and let it go. Whatever it is we encounter in our lives that makes us feel bad about ourselves causing shame, insecurity, fear, etc. we have to be very careful not to turn it on ourselves in a negative, or abusive way. When we feel hurt, we feel vulnerable, and almost immediately a thought can pop up telling us we're not good enough, or that it's our fault that something unpleasant or unfortunate has happened to us. It's so easy to assume responsibility for something that's gone wrong when it might not even be our fault, or that it was out of our control.

Many people immediately blame themselves when something negative happens to them. The end of a relationship or marriage is a perfect example of how someone can go into a complete downward spiral of negativity, thinking that it's their fault that it failed or ended, and the very thought of thinking that you're a "failure" is what dominates your mind. The problem with that is if you don't confront or challenge the very first negative thought you have that wants to throw you under the bus, the next thing you know you can literally feel like you are being run over by all of the negative or abusive thoughts you have until you tell them to stop, by confronting and challenging them with the *Says Who?* method. If you allow for abusive thoughts then you are siding with the abuser, and that person can be yourself just as easily as it can be someone else.

## The Bully Phenomenon

Lately, it seems that we're hearing more and more disturbing stories about young people who are committing suicide because they have been tormented or bullied by someone, causing them to feel hopelessness and deep despair, and no other alternative than to end their life. What's so terribly sad about this horrible, seemingly widespread phenomenon that seems almost epidemic is that so many of these young, innocent people who are victims of prejudice, judgment and hate cannot protect themselves from this harm or abuse. That is, not only are they unable to stand up to the bully and the mean, hateful things being thrown at them, but they also can't stop hearing those very things repeated over and over in their minds later on. In other words, they can't turn off the negative, destructive thoughts reverberating in their mind when they're by themselves because they have taken on those thoughts as true and real. That's why it's so imperative to challenge these thoughts so they don't have power over you for days, months, or even years.

Imagine not being able to turn off those vicious, degrading thoughts someone has planted in your mind. Along with the constant outside bullying, which only reinforces how awful you feel you are and how much you should hate yourself, it just becomes too overwhelming to endure the torment and misery, and you will do anything you can to stop or end your anguish—including suicide.

I can't emphasize enough how important it is for people to know that they do not have to accept anyone's mean and hurtful words, judgments or opinions of them, and that someone else's negative thoughts do not belong to you. It's equally important to know "you are not your negative thoughts," especially as they are trying to pull you down and destroy you. Even though you may be thinking horrible, demeaning thoughts about yourself, they should not define who you are, and are not your true identity. That's why asking yourself "Says who?" is so important because it's asking "Who is saying this thought in my mind? Is it me or did someone else plant this thought in my mind and I accepted it as real and true?"

*Remember, those negative, critical thoughts are not real!*
*They are a temporary distortion of how you see yourself,*
*and if you challenge the thoughts that are causing that*
*distortion, you will see that they are not real or true.*

Asking yourself "Am I in control of this thought?" lets you see how you are not in control of it if it's having such a negative effect on you. You are the one that should always be in control of destructive thoughts instead of allowing them to control you. Ask yourself a follow-up question: "Who's in charge here. Is it me, or is it my mind?" The mind is a powerful thing, and you need to be in control of it and the thoughts that occupy it or it can wreak havoc, and have you believing all sorts of distorted ideas.

We do not come into the world thinking negative, critical, demeaning or destructive thoughts. They are learned and accepted as real and true based on the negative or difficult experiences we've had and how we've interpreted them, or because of what other people tell us, and we've accepted them as real and true. Prejudice, judgment, and hate are not real. They are harmful projections people put on one another so that they don't have to look at or accept their own unhappiness or hatred of themselves. It's far too easy for people to dump their negative thoughts and feelings on someone else, and make them feel wrong or bad, or blame them as the reason for their troubles or the troubles of the world.

If everyone took responsibility for their own negativity we would have far less prejudice, judgment and hate in the world. But unless people question their own negative and hateful thoughts, and ask themselves, "Who is saying this thought in my mind? Is it me or someone else?" then they will continue to unload their negativity onto someone else, avoiding the truth about themselves they choose not to accept. Everyone has to do their own "mental clean up," and "own their thoughts."

If you can begin with questioning and challenging the very first negative or critical thought that tries to make its way into your mind, wanting you to believe it's true, and challenge it by saying "Says who?" which is saying, "Who is saying this thought to me and why?", you stand a greater chance of not believing it, and therefore not allowing it to tell you who you are. Again, no one should tell you who you are— only you! If you allow yourself to believe what anyone tells you about yourself, especially if it's mean or hateful, then you are turning your back on yourself, and that is the very first step you are taking in allowing your thoughts to control you, which can be destructive or even dangerous.

Why would you want anyone to tell you what you should think or feel about yourself? And more importantly, why would you believe any thought you have that wants to hurt or diminish you, whether it was planted in your mind by you or someone else? Question it! Challenge it! Demand from it what you need, and that is the protection of your well-being, at all costs. If your thoughts aren't providing that for you, get rid of them because *they should work for you*—not you being a slave to them. You should be in control of what *you want to think* and what *you want to believe*, always.

It's important to remember that whenever you are thinking a negative thought, and find yourself at the affect of it—causing you to feel upset or angry—that means that you are allowing that thought to get a rise or reaction out of you. Do you want that? Do you want your negative thoughts to get the best of you? They certainly can, if you let them, and yet they don't have to if you challenge and question them with the *Says who?* method.

As I mentioned in Chapter Two when I discussed how our thoughts influence our lives, the first thing to do when an unpleasant or negative thought comes into your head and threatens to throw you off stride is to **acknowledge** it right away. This will help put you in the **observer mode**, instead of the **reactor mode**. Remember, the three steps are:

1. Acknowledge your thought.
2. Observe it.
3. Do not react to it.

These steps are essential to help you remain in the present moment, with total awareness, so you can be in the right frame of mind to question your negative thoughts without letting them affect you emotionally. By remaining the observer and not the reactor, you can get to the root of why that negative thought is in your mind and begin to release it. That way you are in control of your thought, as opposed to it being in control of you.

And remember: A thought of self-love is a thought of power. Don't give your power away by believing any thought, whether it's your own, or influenced by someone else, that does not completely support the best of who you are. Be kind and loving to yourself like you would a child who needed your care and protection. You deserve the same safekeeping, and mindful attention as much as they would.

*Chapter 12*

# Release And Replace
# Your Negative Thoughts

*You only lose what you cling to.*
**—Buddha**

W hen you question your negative thoughts and realize
that they serve no useful purpose for your well-being
and are most often not even real, you can then decide,
with clarity, if you want to continue harboring them or let them go.
Sometimes people are afraid to let go of a "familiar" thought, even if it's
negative, because they don't know what to replace that thought with.

Negativity has an energy around it that keeps the mind occupied
(as I explained in Chapter Seven, "The Something to Worry About
Thoughts"), and even though it can make you feel anxious, frightened
or insecure, you can mistake that energy as a feeling of importance,

like you're doing something productive like problem solving or being reflective, when in fact you're hosting nothing more than busy uselessness in your mind. What a waste of good mental activity, when you could be filling your mind with thoughts that are productive and beneficial to your intelligence, effectiveness and well-being!

*You could be fulfilling your purpose and doing*
*something meaningful and truly important in your life*
*if you allow for it by simply changing your thoughts.*

Just that idea can cause some to think, "That can't be possible! How can I change my thoughts? They come in and out of my mind all the time—how can I know what I'm going to think?"

While it's true you might not know what a thought will be before you think it (Automatic Thoughts, for example), there should be no doubt about what you can do with those thoughts once you experience them, and not be caught off guard, or even broadsided, if or when they come up, and they will, for sure! Wouldn't you rather know what to do when negative, fear based, or at times, even obliterating thoughts pop into your mind? Not knowing what to do would be like having balls coming at you, and not knowing how to dodge them, or at least be able to put your hands in front of your face to protect it. We need knowledge and tools to use when we have to defend ourselves, and negative thoughts are something you definitely need to defend yourself from by learning how to not accept them and let them go. The *Says Who?* method gives you those tools by teaching you how to confront your negative or fear-based thoughts, and question them, as I said, like you would an intruder on your property who doesn't belong there. It's your job to decide who and what belongs near you, and if it isn't positive or serving your well-being, it doesn't belong anywhere near you.

You have the power to change your negative thoughts so they don't cause you stress or unhappiness by controlling your thinking, and if you can't answer the *Says Who?* question, "Am I in control of this thought?" with a resounding "Yes!" then your negative thought clearly has power over you! Remember—you have the ability to control your thoughts, *always*. Question your thoughts, ask them *Says Who?* and you will come to see how easy it is to **like your thoughts**, **control them** and have them **work for you**, but the key is knowing how to **release** the negative thoughts and **replace** them with positive ones.

## Release and Replace

If your mind is cluttered with too many negative thoughts, a positive thought can feel out of place. By removing a negative thought from your mind, you are making room for a positive one to take its place. Think of it this way: when we're used to something, even if it's not good for us, we accept it often at face value and even expect it because we're accustomed to it. When something different—like a positive thought—pops up, we might not be as receptive to it because it may be unfamiliar, or not in keeping with how we are accustomed to thinking. So we dismiss or reject it and allow a negative one to follow, which undermines or invalidates our initial positive thought.

Example: Say you've been in a bit of a rut for a while and have become used to bad things happening to you, so much so that you start saying things to yourself like, "I'm unlucky," or, "What did I expect? I don't deserve to have something good happen to me." Then, if you suddenly have a thought like, "I feel like something good could happen today," you might follow that with, "but it probably won't because it never does." That's what I describe as conflicting thoughts: one positive, the other negative, which cancels the positive thought out, and you can see how defeating that is. Remember, even if you truly believe you're unlucky because bad things seem to happen to you, unless you **replace** those defeating, pessimistic, "downer" thoughts, your mind will never be able to accept a positive, hopeful one because it will be in direct conflict with the negative belief you have about yourself.

You would think we would prefer all of our thoughts to be positive and productive. Yet old habits run deep, so if having negative thoughts has become a type of thinking you're used to, you need to break that habit by asking yourself the *Says Who?* questions when the first negative thought pops up. This process can begin as soon as you wake up in the morning, which is usually the time when our mind is on automatic, and habitual thoughts start firing in quick succession.

Thoughts like, "I'm unlovable" or "unworthy," can begin your day with a deep feeling of uneasiness and insecurity. If the only thing you think when you look at yourself in the mirror is, "I'm fat" or "ugly" that is a sure recipe for making you feel horrible about yourself the rest of the day, carrying over to when you're driving to work—especially if it's a job you don't like. You might think, "I hate my life," or "I'll never be able to get ahead," giving you a feeling of futility, hopelessness and powerlessness. Maybe those kinds of thoughts feel real for you, but if you don't probe or investigate why you're thinking those thoughts or where they came from in the first place, then you won't feel in control of them, and progress can't be made changing them or reaching the outcome you'd like to achieve: like doing something pro-active about your weight, or finding a solution to changing the job or life you say you hate.

Having a thought like "I'm fat," or "ugly" may be honest, if that's how you feel (though "ugly" is pretty harsh, don't you think?), but unless you challenge those demeaning and defeating thoughts by asking yourself questions like, "Does this thought make feel better?" or, "Does this thought work for me?" (for which the answers are an unequivocal "no"), you will stay stuck in the negative, critical mindset that serves no useful purpose for your well being.

*Remember, if you want to change something you
don't like about yourself, stop calling yourself names.
Again, children do that when they're in the sandbox!*

Negative name-calling does absolutely nothing to help you, and is completely counter-productive to reaching your goals. Asking yourself, "Do I like this thought?" can be very revealing when you find out that you're holding thoughts in your mind *you don't even like!* Who would willingly want to do that? Nobody's forcing you to think negative, critical or diminishing thoughts, so why do it? The *Says Who?* questions are very logical and practical, and will help you see how pointless and useless it is to fill up your mind with nothing other than thoughts that are positive, productive, and serve your well being. Don't settle for anything less to occupy your mind!

*Until you can remove or **release** the opposing negative
thoughts or images in your subconscious and **replace** them
with positive supportive thoughts and images, your conscious
and subconscious mind will always be in a tug-of-war with
one another, making it extremely difficult, if not impossible
for you to realize your dreams, desires and goals.*

When we have a thought in our conscious mind, we usually have an image or a picture that accompanies it. For example, if you tell yourself you would like to eat an apple, the picture or image that most likely pops up in your mind is of a juicy, red or green apple that makes you feel hungry for it. The thought of a rotten apple would never arouse your appetite, so therefore you wouldn't allow for it in your thoughts, nor would it make sense for it to be the image in your mind for something you desire for pleasure. It makes more sense for the image in your mind to match your desire for it. The same would apply again for the desire to lose weight. If you tell yourself you would like to be thinner than you are, imagine seeing yourself as that person and tell yourself that is how you're going to look.

By continuing to see yourself as that person, and repeating over and over again that you "will" realize the optimum weight you desire, you're conscious mind is telling your subconscious what it wants, not the other way around. You are **releasing** or removing the negative image and **replacing** it with the positive one.

Consider this a training of the mind, a *daily practice* of telling yourself who you are and what you want. The only thing the conscious mind asks of you is to commit to what you say you want, and by doing that, you're being very clear about what you're telling your subconscious, which is always absorbing and storing what you think. Remember, you're in the driver's seat of your thoughts, navigating where you want to go, so be clear about where that is. No mixed messages! As I said before, the subconscious takes its orders from *you*. If you tell it: "I am going to lose $x$ lbs. because I want to, and I see myself as that person and it makes me happy to be who I really am," your subconscious will believe it. Remember the apple image. If you want one, it isn't rotten when you picture it, so why would you picture yourself as anything less than desirable? See yourself as you'd like yourself to be, and continue seeing yourself like that by holding that image in your mind. Your desire needs to match the image you have, otherwise the conflicting messages in your conscious and subconscious will result in a "tug-of-war," and the negative side will always try to dominate and win.

I'll give you another example. I had a client who had been seeing a woman for a few years and he would not commit to marrying her. He told her he wanted to marry her, but when push came to shove, he couldn't pull the trigger. Obviously there was something holding him back from taking the big step, causing frustration for his girlfriend. He said he loved and cared for her, but her frustration with him was starting to make him feel uncomfortable and pressured. Clearly, there was something keeping him from fully committing to her, and that's what we needed to find out.

When I asked him if he wanted to marry her, he gave me a definitive "yes," but when I asked him what was stopping him, he said something vague like, "I'm not ready," and shrugged. At our next session it was clear his ambivalence about marrying his girlfriend was taking its toll, and the relationship was suffering.

"Close your eyes," I said to him, and asked him to tell me what image comes up for him when he thinks about marrying his girlfriend. His eyes were only closed a minute before he exclaimed, "Oh man!"

"What image came to your mind?" I asked.

He opened his eyes. "I saw my brother!"

"Why do you think your brother came up as your image for marrying your girlfriend?"

He told me the story of how his older brother who he really looked up to got married straight out of high school because he got his girlfriend pregnant. The marriage turned out to be a disaster, and his brother, who wanted to be a doctor and go to medical school, got entangled in an ugly divorce, and ended up not going after his dream of becoming a doctor. He blamed it on a terrible decision he made to marry the woman he got pregnant. He saw his brother suffer, and become embittered by the wrong choice he had made. He never married again.

Bingo! We had gotten to the exact reason for my client's problem. He had taken on his brother's bad experience and let that be his own idea or "image" of what getting married could turn out to be—a mistake, or better yet, a disaster. In his mind, his image, which was negative, is in direct opposition to the very positive thing he desires, which is to marry the woman he loves.

"But that happened to your brother, not to you," I said.

"I know, but it could happen to me too," he said. "It's possible."

"Can you see how you're holding the picture of your brother's failed marriage in your mind when the thought of making a commitment to your girlfriend comes up?"

"I do. It does seem kind of crazy to me since it happened to my brother so long ago, but I can't seem to rid myself of him saying marriage isn't worth it."

"You've been holding that thought and image in your mind for a long time," I said. "That's how long we can carry around a thought we believe is true."

"I don't want to picture my brother when it comes to marrying the woman I'm in love with, or think that it will end up being a mistake. That doesn't seem fair to her or me."

"It isn't fair to you or your girlfriend because that's your brother's belief, not yours," I said, "which means it's not your original thought. You've taken his negative thought on as your own, and turned it into a belief that you've accepted as true, and it's affecting your relationship. Can you see that?"

"Yeah, I really can," he said with a deep sigh. It was as if the proverbial light bulb went off. This was his "aha moment, " realizing that he is not his brother, and not destined to repeat his fate, just like I was not destined to have the unfortunate fate of my sister. He married his girlfriend a few months later.

By having my client picture what getting married looked like in his mind, he was able to see an image, his brother, and how it was in direct opposition to what he really wanted, which was to marry his girlfriend. That, coupled with him realizing that his brother's negative belief in marriage had become his too, making it not his own "original" thought, helped him shift his thinking, which then changed the image he held in his mind about marriage. In other words, it went from a negative image to a positive one, and that's what you need to hold in your mind's eye when you picture the very thing you really want. My client needed to

**release** his brother's thought, which he did, and **replace** it with his own positive thought, which was, "I'm ready to marry the woman I love."

The process of releasing a negative thought, which, as we've seen, can create a negative image in your mind that can be in direct opposition to a desire you have (like losing weight or committing to a relationship) requires that you acknowledge that you are holding that negative thought or image in your mind, and that you want to replace it with something positive that supports your desire. You can't replace a negative thought or image unless you are really ready to let it go. Another way to find out if you're ready is by asking yourself if you're also ready to let any feelings—such as unworthiness or feeling unlovable that you might have around those negative thoughts or images also go. One of the main reasons we hold onto negative thoughts about ourselves is because we might not feel that we deserve something better in our lives.

However, while it may feel natural to give in to these types of feelings, I'd like you to consider another idea: Allow what you're feeling to be with you. Welcome it. Acknowledge it. It is only when we let that feeling surface that we can then **observe** it, **identify** it and then be able to **release** it and **replace** it with a more positive, productive thought, which creates an equally productive and positive feeling. Then, once you've acknowledged and identified the feeling, ask yourself these questions:

- *Could I let this feeling go?*
- *Am I willing to let this feeling go?*
- *If so, can I do it now?*

For every thought or feeling that is negative or self-critical, pick it apart. Break it down. If you feel you're unworthy or unlovable, challenge that thought, almost like you're saying to it: "Oh yeah? Says Who!?" It's like you're asking it to prove itself to you before you're so quick to believe it—and you should. You have the power, and are in control to do this. As I've said, your thoughts should be **working for you, not you working for them,** and you can turn those negative, annoying thoughts around at any time by first confronting and challenging them, and then making the decision to release them, and allow the positive ones to take their place.

Say you're feeling unlovable. The following shows you how to challenge those thoughts using the *Says who?* method with a response:

| Question | Response |
|---|---|
| *Says Who?* | I am saying I'm unlovable. Why do I believe that? |
| *Did I hear someone say this thought before?* | My wife told me I was more loveable when we got married. After my divorce, I felt unlovable. |
| *Do I like this thought?* | I don't like thinking that I'm unlovable. |
| *Does this thought make me feel better?* | Thinking I'm unlovable makes me feel bad about myself. |
| *Does this thought work for me?* | Thinking I'm unlovable makes me insecure. No, it's not working for me. |
| *Am I in control of this thought?* | The thought that I'm unlovable is always in the back of my mind. I wish it wasn't there controlling me. |
| *Do I want to keep this thought or let it go?* | I don't want to keep thinking that I'm unlovable, and want to go back to feeling that I am lovable. I want to let it go. |

*Remember, when you remove a negative thought from your mind, you make room for a positive one to replace it, and that positive thought can create a positive image to match it, which can manifest your reality.*

Make some room for those positive thoughts!

## Chapter 13

# Action Thoughts

*Thought is the blossom, language the bud, action the fruit behind it.*
**—Ralph Waldo Emerson**

Remember, whatever you tell yourself gets stored in your subconscious, which, as I described, is like a basement where all of your memories of your experiences are kept. It believes everything you tell it as true and real, unless you change your thoughts and tell it otherwise. Thinking negative or judgmental thoughts without challenging them with the *Says Who?* method can keep them stuck in your mind, which does nothing useful to help you get "unstuck" from your negative beliefs about yourself. That's why, as I've said before, it's imperative that you question and challenge those types of thoughts with the *Says Who?* method as soon as they pop up. Then, once you've challenged them, you can change those negative thoughts from being something that tears you down into something positive that builds you up and serves your well-being.

> *If you want to change a negative thought into something productive and useful, turn it into an* **Action Thought,** *which is a positive thought that tells your subconscious* **what you want to do** *proactively instead of telling yourself something negative* **that you think you are,** *which is name calling and useless.*

For example, if you tell yourself you're stupid, or fat, or untalented (or anything that is demeaning or diminishing), your subconscious will believe you—and why wouldn't it since it's taking direction and orders from you. But if you tell yourself that you want to be better at something, or lose weight, or express your creativity, your thoughts are then motivated by *action*, which will stimulate or inspire you to take responsibility for what you want to change about yourself, and get you started in the right direction. *Action Thoughts take your desire and literally move you forward towards realizing your goal.* Think of it as the fire under your seat that gets you going.

But before you use those Action Thoughts to motivate you into "doing," it's important that you begin with questioning your negative thoughts with the *Says Who?* method first so you can discover the **origin** of those thoughts, the **reasons** behind them, and know if they are **real** or not. Once you complete these questions and are clear as to why you are thinking any thought that is negative and does not serve your well-being, you can then try the following Action Thought technique to change any ongoing negative thoughts into proactive thoughts.

| Examples of changing a negative thought into an Action Thought: | |
| --- | --- |
| **Negative Thought** | **Action Thought** |
| I'm never going to get a job. | **I will** look for a job tomorrow. |
| I'm going to end up alone. | **I will** put myself out there so I can meet someone. |
| I'm going to end up with no money. | **I will** plan better for my future and find ways to save my money so I will be secure later on in my life. |
| I'm not in good shape. | **I will** start taking care of myself by eating well and exercising so I can get into better shape. |
| I don't have good friends who are there for me. | **I will** make an effort to make friends who I can rely on, and be there for them too when they need me. |
| I'm uninteresting and boring. | **I will** get interested in more diverse things that I can share with other people so they won't find me one dimensional or boring. |
| I'm unsuccessful at love. | **I will** be successful at love. Just because I've had some unpleasant or difficult relationships doesn't mean I'm unsuccessful at love. |
| I'm a weak person. | **I will** focus on my strengths instead of my weaknesses to remind myself that I am strong in ways that are important. |

| I'm unattractive. | **I will** focus on ways to make myself look more attractive and appealing rather than being critical. Anyone can be more attractive with a little effort and so can I. |
|---|---|
| I'm not really good at anything in particular. | **I will** focus on something I have the potential to be good at, and make an effort to get better at it, and not criticize myself in the process. |

These are all examples of how you can turn your negative thoughts into positive Action Thoughts. As we've seen in previous chapters, a thought that is negative, judgmental or critical is useless—it does nothing other than stay negative in your mind, and often causes more negative thoughts to come up. But if you can turn it into an Action Thought, you are changing a negative thought (that tells you what you're "not" or what you "can't" do) into what you *can* and *will* do. Thoughts like "I'm not, " can suddenly be, "I am!"; "I can't," becomes "I can!" or "I will!"

From there you can expand your Action Thought into declaring whatever it is you want to do or accomplish—"**I am** going to lose weight," or "**I can** finish my project," or "**I will** be open to a relationship, etc. An Action Thought takes a negative thought and turns it completely around. Once you get familiar with the technique, you will see how it propels you into positive action.

If you really want to do something or get something done, it makes sense that you would think a thought that motivates you to do it, right? By asking yourself the *Says Who?* question, "Does this thought work for me?" you will know if your thought is helping you "do" as opposed to "not do" what you say you want to, and clearly if you answer the question "Does this thought make me feel better?" and you answer with "No," then you can't turn the thought that isn't making you feel better about yourself into an Action Thought, and go after what you want.

Action Thoughts motivate your desire, so if you turn a negative thought like "I'm fat," into an Action Thought like, "**I will** lose weight," you are telling your subconscious what you want to do. And remember, it takes its direction and orders from you.

The reason why goals are often not met is that they are usually not supported and backed by Action Thoughts. You need to stay consistent with your Action Thoughts to achieve the kind of outcome or result you're hoping for. For instance, if you tell yourself that you want to lose weight, you need to be not only disciplined with what you eat, but also with the thoughts that are supporting you and motivating you to continue **daily**. It's very easy to find yourself running out of steam if your daily thoughts aren't supporting your desire, and you can find yourself unmotivated to stick to it because your thoughts aren't fueling you properly to continue reaching toward your goal. The only way to guard against this is to keep your Action Thoughts—the type of thoughts that move you into positive action, as opposed to *distraction* or *destruction*—constant. Action thoughts move you out, and literally push you forward to reach the goals you want to achieve. *Says Who?* supports this by helping eliminate the self defeating thoughts that often are not even real, and direct you to your correct Action Thoughts.

Diets are a good example of how frustrating and often disappointing it can be when you can't reach your goal because of feeling defeated. Many people are quick to give up when it's not going how they expect it to, or have a little setback, but what makes a diet successful is not just your *desire* to lose weight and your initial *commitment* to it. Success requires that you have a *daily mental discipline* of keeping your thoughts in Action Mode, meaning they have to keep supporting what you want by telling yourself what to do, e.g. "I'm watching my calories today," or "I'm going to walk a little longer, " or "I'm going to exercise a little harder." The name of the game is consistency, and that means telling yourself positive, pro-active thoughts every day, and not allowing yourself to slip into old habits of thinking, such as negative or critical thoughts like "I'm still so fat," or "I still hate how I look," or "I just can't do this, so why bother."

Having positive, supportive Action Thoughts on Monday, Wednesday and Friday, but not on the other days of the week, isn't going to help you reach your goal either. Even if you do have a setback day where you aren't feeling as motivated, and maybe even go off your diet, do not beat yourself up with harsh, demeaning words! That can cause you to give up, and then feel bad about yourself that you did, which will only make you feel worse, causing the negative, critical thoughts to start all over again. If you slip, it's in the past; don't dwell on it. Move forward in your mind-set by saying "**I will** start my diet again." You can jump right into using your supportive Action Thoughts whenever you need to start over. A beginning is always a fresh start, and there's no need to look back to what you didn't do yesterday. "I didn't" becomes "I did." Today is about "Action!"

Remember, if you have a temporary setback, or slip up reaching your goal, be it losing weight or whatever you desire to do, the minute a negative, critical thought comes up, perform these three steps first:

1. Acknowledge it.
2. Observe it.
3. Do not react to it.

By not being reactive to the self-defeating "I can't" thoughts, you will be open and ready to change them to "I can" or "I will." So again, in the case of losing weight, instead of saying, "I'm never going to lose weight," you *acknowledge* it as a negative thought and *observe* yourself having that feeling, which will then help you to *not react negatively* to it. Then, because you prepared yourself by working the *Says Who?* method, to identify the source of your negative self-judgment, you can move forward with an Action Thought and tell yourself something like, "I'm back on track to get my weight down," and believe it. And even if days or weeks go by where you've gone off track, remember, you can jump back in at any time with an Action Thought.

This *Action Thought* technique should be able to help you when you find yourself slipping into old negative habits of thinking while you're in the midst of trying to stay positive on your course to reach a goal. It should not take the place of the *Says Who?* method, which is essential in helping you get to the origin of your negative thought so that you can first identify it, find out why you're thinking it, and if it's real or not. It's a supplement to it, designed to help you move closer to achieving your desires.

Remember, until you get to the root of your negative thought, you can't change it. Once you do, you can turn it into an Action Thought to realize your goal and manifest what you want.

## Chapter 14

# Change Old Negative Beliefs
# Into Current Positive Beliefs

*If you don't change your beliefs, your life
will be like this forever. Is that good news?*
**—W. Somerset Maugham**

A s we now know, our negative beliefs get stored in our subconscious, and until we change them, they will remain there. Always try and keep in mind, if you can, that whatever you tell yourself stays in that "thought basement" of yours. It's also good to remember the agreement between your conscious and subconscious mind, as far as how they work together in tandem. Sometimes we forget the dual function they serve, and we can get sloppy and lazy with the thoughts we're feeding ourselves, but our subconscious is standing by like a dutiful soldier, ready to obey our every command.

By not challenging your negative thoughts when they come up is allowing them to seep right into your subconscious, and if you can think of it like a sponge that's ready to soak up every bit of negativity you have for it—it will. I'm hoping, however, that after you've used the *Says Who?* method, and gotten a sense of what it's like to stop a negative thought right in its tracks, that you'll be ready to let go of some of those old negative beliefs you're holding onto, and replace them with current positive thoughts that can be stored in your subconscious as your **"new beliefs."** And even if you feel that your negative thoughts outweigh the positive ones you have right now, I can assure you that if you have just a few "sweet" thoughts floating around, they can out do your negative ones pretty quickly, if you just give it a try.

Here's how it works: Think of an old negative belief you've been holding onto—let's say, something like, "I'm never going to have the life I really want." Ask yourself "Says who? Who is saying I'll never have the life I really want?" You can answer with "I am saying that," which lets you know you are taking responsibility for having that thought (owning it). Now think of a positive current thought you have, which could be something like, "I want to travel more." You may think that those two thoughts have nothing to do with each other, but if you can put your focus on your positive thought -- that you "want to travel more," it can easily be turned into a "belief" by saying "I **will** travel more," while the old belief, "I'll never have the life I really want" can be dissolved by a current desire you have, which is to travel.

You can then say to yourself "I am letting go of the belief that I'll never have the life I really want," and change it to a new belief, "**I will** travel more," which can only add to creating the life you say you want. This takes your current "positive" belief and turns it into an Action Thought, and the "I'm not" or "I can't" or "I won't" becomes "I am, I can, and I will." And if you asked yourself the question, "Does this thought make me feel better," once you've changed your thought, there's no doubt you would answer it with, "Yes, this thought makes me feel better."

It's important to acknowledge when a thought improves how you feel, which will help you detect immediately the feeling of "good energy" that comes with a positive thought, and the "bad energy" you feel with a negative thought. Getting good at feeling the difference between those two energies can help you determine if there's something going on with your thoughts that you need to address. Remember, our thoughts create our feelings, so if you can connect a negative thought with an uncomfortable feeling in your body, you will become less tolerant of it, and be that much more inclined to change your negative thoughts. The goal for using the *Says Who?* method is to connect you—mind, body and spirit—in the best way possible, so that everything is flowing and working just right in your **entire** being.

By questioning and challenging your **old negative beliefs**, you have the opportunity to change them into **new positive beliefs**. It's a good idea to update your beliefs and make sure they are in synch with your thoughts:

**Positive Thoughts = Positive Beliefs**
**Negative Thoughts = Negative Beliefs**

There has to be a cohesive exchange between your conscious and subconscious mind if you want to get them speaking the same language. It's like that saying, "The left hand needs to know what the right hand is doing." It's all about good communication. But if you're still accepting of your old negative beliefs and not willing to let them go, you can't "update them" with your current positive thoughts, which you have every opportunity to turn into positive, productive, "current" beliefs. The negative one's go out, and the new positive ones go in. It's really that simple. When you accept it, so does your subconscious. Here's how it works:

**Accepting negative thoughts = Keeping negative beliefs**
**Changing negative thoughts to positive thoughts =**
**Changing negative beliefs into positive beliefs**

*Some of our old negative beliefs can be left over from when we were children—that's how far back they can go!*

When we're children we can be called many critical or unkind things, and not just by our peers, but by siblings, parents and others—people we love, look up to or admire. And sometimes what they say to us it isn't necessarily meant to be hurtful, but to emphasize a point, like telling you that you're forgetful or accident prone, or overly dramatic, etc.

"Absentminded" and "clumsy" or "dramatic" are names that some of us grew up hearing about ourselves and have accepted as true. But if you don't question or challenge those beliefs about yourself today, when you've obviously grown and matured, then you're holding onto an old negative belief that was influenced or instilled in you by someone else, and haven't **"updated"** it. Maybe you were forgetful or scattered as a child, but *you were a child!* Most children are that way, but now that you're an adult, that thought might not hold true anymore, and yet you have held onto it as a "belief" about yourself.

If you can connect a negative thought you have to someone else having said it to you, and recognize that it was not your **original** thought about yourself, but something someone once told you that you are, you might want to inquire if it holds true today. That's why asking yourself "Have I heard someone say this thought before?" helps you get to the origin of your thought to find out if it was someone else's thought or opinion of you that you took on as your own.

In the case of being "absentminded" or "clumsy," ask yourself, *Says Who?* which means: "Who said I was absent minded or clumsy?" and "Am I calling myself those names because I believe it's true?" And whether it's you that is saying it, or someone else said it about you, ask yourself if you believe you still are something you were called at one time. If you no longer are accident prone or forgetful, you can let go of that belief about yourself because it no longer holds true anymore, and can tell yourself that this is not who you are **today**.

*Why hold onto old beliefs that other people have placed on you if it doesn't pertain to who you are in the present, and is inaccurate?*

Thinking that you're stupid is a thought many people grew up feeling, or have thought about themselves at some point in their lives. Having that opinion either comes from someone telling you that you are, or because you compared yourself to someone else and perceived them as better or smarter than you at something.

I had a client who grew up feeling not very smart. When I asked him if someone made him feel that way, he said, "Yes, a teacher in elementary school." It wasn't until years later when he was a young adult and took a series of IQ and aptitude tests that he found out that he, in fact, was very intelligent. He held the belief about himself that he was stupid for most of his childhood, and it was an automatic thought that would come up frequently for him whenever something triggered that feeling, like feeling anxiety about a test, or performing well at sports. Although that teacher never actually called him "stupid," he felt he was by the way she treated him, and he then labeled himself "dumb". After he was tested, and realized how intelligent he actually was, he then felt confident to challenge that belief about himself, but admitted that it was hard to fully let go of a belief he held about himself for so long.

He became a successful writer, but had he not challenged his belief that he was stupid because someone once made him feel that he was, he never would have gone on to prove that thought inaccurate and not true.

Unless a thought like "I'm stupid" can be backed up by evidence or proof, you might want to question and probe that thought further with the *Says Who?* questions to find out if it's true or inaccurate. For instance, here's how we used the method together to challenge the "I'm stupid" thought, which had turned into a belief:

| Question | Response |
|---|---|
| *Says who?* | I am telling myself that I'm stupid. |
| *Have I heard someone say this thought before?* | My teacher made me feel stupid. She used to say things that didn't make me feel very smart. |
| *Do I like this thought?* | I don't like thinking that I'm stupid. |
| *Does this thought make me feel better?* | No. Thinking that I'm stupid makes me feel really bad. |
| *Does this thought work for me?* | Thinking that I'm stupid makes me feel like I can't do certain things. It doesn't make me feel confident or work for me in a positive way at all. |
| *Am I in control of this thought?* | Sometimes when I feel challenged, I think that I'm stupid, and that thought plays over and over again in my mind like I'm not in control of it. |

| Do I want to keep this thought or let it go? | I've wanted to let go of the thought that I'm stupid for a very long time. I'm ready to. |
|---|---|

By asking yourself these fundamental questions, like he did, it will become more clear to you how holding onto a negative thought like "I'm stupid" serves no useful purpose at all, other than being self-critical and perpetuating a belief about yourself that may not be accurate or based on truth. As I've said before, these thoughts usually stem from a distorted perception you have of yourself because of either something someone once said to you or because you compared yourself to someone else that you perceived as smarter than you.

Feeling less than or "not good enough" is an unnatural state to be in. We don't come into the world that way. Someone or something causes us to feel less than or inferior, and we allow for it. Most of us have experienced, and can even remember the first time someone said something that made us feel bad about ourselves. Kids say mean things to one another all the time, and it's usually as early as elementary school when we experience that feeling for the first time that we're not good enough or unworthy, unlovable, or even stupid.

The reason we accept feeling less than and believe thinking that way is "normal" is because we don't question or challenge the accuracy or truth of what we tell ourselves or what others have told us about ourselves. That's because when we hear or feel those sentiments as children we don't yet have the tools or awareness to question our thoughts cognitively, or have the intellectual ability to know how our thoughts work. If you don't know how to prove whether a thought is true, which the *Says Who?* method helps you do, then it's easy to accept a negative thought as real, and allow for it to be an old belief about yourself that you're still holding onto.

Unless you change your negative thoughts by questioning them, you will accept them as true and real, and they remain a part of your belief system and can stay that way your whole life. How wonderful it would be if we were able to question our negative thoughts or beliefs about ourselves when we're children and stand up to them, knowing they weren't true. But children are sensitive, vulnerable, gullible, and more likely to believe what's told to them. It takes a pretty strong, confident child to say something like, "I don't believe you!" and stand up to someone calling them mean names. The old saying "Sticks and stones may break my bones but names can never harm me," is a way to resist negative, hurtful words, but that saying is dated. A more current way to stand up for yourself is by declaring, "Says who?" when a negative thought pops up, which, in its own way, is like saying "I'm not believing or accepting what you say because I don't have to!"

But even once childhood is left behind, many people grow up and still believe the negative thoughts they have because they haven't challenged them or changed their beliefs about themselves, and therefore walk around with low self-esteem. For someone who has a low opinion about themselves, or feels insecure about something, it can be hard for them to receive or accept a compliment or any kind of praise. Their negative belief about themselves is so deeply ingrained in their thinking that no matter how much you compliment them or tell them they're good or worthy or lovable, they just can't let it in and accept it. They can't let it penetrate the power of what they believe about themselves, and your positive words cannot convince them differently.

That is why no matter what someone says to you, even if they tell you that you're great or special, unless you can change what you fundamentally believe about yourself, and the negative thoughts that support that belief, you can't change that negative belief for the better. How many times have we heard a successful actor or celebrity talk about how insecure they are or unworthy they feel of the accolades they receive? Those revelations are by no means rare; in fact they practically built the careers of Madonna and Oprah Winfrey.

Madonna famously admitted, "I think my biggest flaw is my insecurity. I'm plagued with insecurities 24/7." It's hard to believe someone like Madonna can be at the mercy of insecurity like the rest of us, yet she's become incredibly successful in spite of them.

Oprah is another example. She has not only turned her insecurities into self-acceptance, she has also built an empire on that notion in the process. She's admitted to being "obsessed with weight," and has struggled with it for a long time, but finally got to a place where she realized "you are not the shape of your body." That realization means that, to her, her identity is not attached to her weight, and indicates that how she feels about herself is more positive than negative. That takes mental discipline to not allow your negative thoughts and beliefs about yourself to dictate who you are, and how you feel about yourself.

But, for some people, their insecurities plague them to the point where they can't transcend them, and are unable to reach their goals or realize their dreams as a result. The solution is not to allow your negative thoughts to keep supporting a negative belief about yourself. Ask yourself the *Says Who?* questions so you can find out if your negative thoughts:

1. Are your own.
2. Someone else's.
3. Likeable.
4. Encouraging.
5. Working for you.
6. Controlling you.
7. Worth keeping.

It's important to question our thoughts and beliefs regularly so we can keep them "updated" to reflect who we are today, and not who we were at another time in our lives. By doing so, we can know which thoughts are still lingering around in our mind that don't serve our well being, and decide if we want to keep them or finally let them go. When we keep thoughts and beliefs that are not positive or productive, but negative and counter-productive, it can throw our whole thinking process off kilter, and that's when we doubt ourselves, and fall back into old patterns of thinking. Find out if you are holding onto "old negative beliefs" that are getting in the way of your current "positive thoughts" that want to thrive successfully in your mind. The whole idea is to keep your thoughts **"current" (positive),** and do away with the ones that are **"old" (negative).**

Remember, who you are today, isn't who you once were, and you no longer have to live in the shadow of who you were before, or at any other time other than the present. You can attach any new "positive" name or description of yourself that you feel best describes who you are today. It's all about declaring: **"I am,"** and doing away with who you aren't anymore. You define who you are. Nobody else does.

*Chapter 15*

# Thoughts of Forgiveness, Compassion & Love

*Compassion, forgiveness, these are the real, ultimate sources of power for peace and success in life.*
**—Dalai Lama**

When we hold onto negative thoughts about things that have happened to us in the past, it keeps us stuck there, and unable to free ourselves of a memory that was unpleasant or hurtful. The problem with holding onto thoughts connected to something or someone we have negative feelings towards is that whenever we think of it or them, it evokes a similar reaction in us, which not only keeps us at the affect of what happened in the past, but also keeps us a **reactor** instead of an **observer.**

What this does is it makes you feel like you're reliving the same thing over and over again every time you think of it, and the outcome you experience will be exactly as before, and nothing will change for you in the process. The reason for that is that you haven't changed the fundamental thought around something that has happened in your past, and until you "update" that thought, as I explained before, it will be as alive for you today as it was when it happened. By asking yourself the Says Who? questions, you are shining a light on the thoughts that no longer work for you, and if you're ready to release them once and for all, the method will help you do it.

If you ask yourself even two of the seven questions: "Does this thought work for me?" or "Does this thought make me feel better?" and the answer for you is "No," then you might want to consider replacing your thought about that person, or the incident that happened, with thoughts of **Forgiveness, Compassion** and **Love**, which might seem like a tall order for you, especially if you're not used to thinking thoughts of that nature, but maybe it's time that you give it a try.

Letting go of negative thoughts, and replacing them with thoughts that are more about acceptance and kindness, instead of resentment and blame, allows for your heart to open more, and heal the unpleasant or hurtful memories you might still be holding onto. One of the most important *Says Who?* questions to ask yourself if you're holding onto negative thoughts from your past is "Do I want to keep this thought or let it go?" You have to find out if you are finally ready to let go of the negative thought that still keeps the unpleasant or hurtful memory very much alive in your mind. Unless you change your negative thought for good, you know that it will just stay stored in your subconscious as a belief, and even if that thought isn't always conscious in your mind, when something triggers it, it will only set you off, causing you to relive your past again and again. What this means is that you are not in control of your thought, it still controls you, hence the necessary question, "Am

I in control of this thought?" which clearly you're not if you are unable to let it go, and that's why it's so important that it be changed on a deep, fundamental level for good.

If you can rise above your disappointment or hurt "feelings" and instead be more magnanimous, that is, generous of spirit or big-hearted, it will be easier for you to hold thoughts of **forgiveness, compassion** and **love** towards anyone or anything that you feel caused you unhappiness instead of holding any ill feelings towards them. What you will gain instead is your heart and mind working in synch, rather than your mind at the mercy of an old negative belief that no longer works for you. By expanding your mind to transform your thoughts, you no longer have to be at the mercy of what once was, but instead live your life thinking about **"what is"** today. *The Says Who?* method will always keep you in the present, and if you happen to think about something unpleasant from your past, by plugging it into the seven Says Who? questions, your default place will be to release any thoughts of anger or resentment, and replace them with thoughts that serve your well-being, and give you a feeling of wholeness, as well as achieving closure from your past. Thoughts of **forgiveness, compassion** and **love** will always transcend negative thoughts, and not allow for baser thoughts to thrive in your mind. The *Says Who?* method will help you elevate your mindset, and not allow for it to be stuck at a lower level of non-forgiveness. When you function from this productive, more conscious way of thinking, you will find that you have much more room in your heart for forgiveness of yourself and others.

Our minds and thoughts are tremendously powerful, and as I've explained throughout the book, they create our reality, and each day you can decide what that reality is for yourself. I encourage you to always try and make a habit of replacing your negative thoughts with positive ones, but what I'm suggesting also is to go even further, and *think of yourself as the architect of your mind*. What kind of thoughts are you constructing? What do you want them to reflect of you? What images do they conjure up? Ultimately, what are the thoughts you choose to occupy your mind of "today?" Are they made up of thoughts that are about **forgiveness, compassion** and **love**, or dominated by negative thoughts from your past that are about resentment and being unforgiving? If they are, ask yourself "Says who?" which means, "who is saying this thought in my mind?" Is it you, and if so, which type of thoughts do you think would ultimately make you feel better, hence the question, "Does this thought make me feel better?" Thoughts of **forgiveness, compassion** and **love** will always make us feel better than holding onto any negative thoughts from our past. Yesterday has come and gone. Release those past negative thoughts, and allow for the positive ones that support how you want your heart to feel today. Those are the thoughts worth listening to and believing.

# PART III

# Transform
# Your Thoughts

*Man's mind, once stretched by a new idea,*
*never regains its original dimensions.*
**—Oliver Wendell Holmes**

*Chapter 16*

# Mindfulness: A New
# Way Of Thinking

*If you are depressed, you are living in the past. If you are anxious, you are living in the future. If you are at peace, you are living in the present.*

**—Lao Tzu**

This final section of the book is called "Transform Your Thoughts" because it will give you the tools to do just that. While Section One told us how our thoughts worked, and Section Two helped us identify our thoughts and know them better, this section is where the work begins. I will show you how to incorporate the *Says Who?* method into a daily practice, so that you are more present, aware and observant of your thoughts, and thus able to handle the stresses, obstacles and negativity that invariably pop up in life. Before you get started, I want you to think about how Mindfulness plays an important role in understanding ourselves better, and is such an integral part of this process.

When we are in the present moment of our lives with total awareness, we are being "Mindful." In a **mindful state,** our thoughts tend to be more accepting of ourselves and what is, rather than what isn't or what could be. Most of our thoughts that take us out of the present moment are either occupied with the past, which we cannot change, or the future, which is unknown to us until it occurs. That's why when you live your life focusing on what is happening right in that exact moment—**the present**—you can be that much more aware when your thoughts are trying to take you out of the present, and pull you in the direction of the past or future.

"Mindfulness," which comes from the Buddhist tradition, and is "considered to be of great importance on the path to enlightenment" is having an awareness of the reality of things in the present moment. The *Says Who?* method helps keep us in the present moment so that we can focus on our thoughts when they are negative or fearful, and by being the "observer" and not the "reactor" of our thoughts; we can maintain a "calm awareness," as we remove the negative thoughts from our mind.

*Says Who?* not only helps you be in the present moment by asking yourself seven specifically designed questions for any thought that disrupts your positive and productive state of mind(fulness), but it also helps you stay in the present moment with a sharper awareness of all of your thoughts constantly coming and going in your mind. If Mindfulness is being aware of our thoughts, making the *Says Who?* method a daily practice will help keep that mindfulness consistent.

By asking yourself "Says who?" when a negative or fearful thought comes up, you are confronting the realness or truth of it, head on. It's like saying to a negative thought: "I want to know *in this moment* what you want from me, and why you are trying to take me out of a positive, present state of mind, causing me worry, doubt or fear." Just as easily as the tides can turn, at any given moment in our day, so can our thoughts, and we can be taken out of a positive state of mind. As we know, it's not always easy to stay in the present moment and maintain the mental discipline to keep ourselves in a calm, peaceful and confident state of being. *Says Who?* gives you seven solid questions to ask yourself when you are being pulled out of the moment by negative or fearful thoughts:

1. Says who?
2. Have I heard someone say this thought before?
3. Do I like this thought?
4. Does this thought make me feel better?
5. Does this thought work for me?
6. Am I in control of this thought?
7. Do I want to keep this thought or let it go?

These questions remind us that *we have a right to stay in the present moment*, thinking positive, productive thoughts, and deserve to be calm, peaceful, and non judgmental of ourselves and others. We don't need to accept a state of mind that is less than positive, or think anything that diminishes us, and does not serve our well-being. Without questioning your negative thoughts, however, it's far too easy to forget that you are in charge of your thoughts at all times and determine how you want to feel, when negative or fearful thoughts enter your mind.

*Says Who?* will help keep you mindful of them, and by being mindful, you have the awareness to question any thought that interrupts or conflicts with your state of being. These two work together beautifully:

**Mindfulness = Thinking With Awareness**

By questioning your thoughts, you will continue to be more mindful of any thought that is not keeping you in the present moment in a positive state.

*Chapter 17*

# Your Daily Discipline

*A disciplined mind leads to happiness,*
*and an undisciplined mind leads to suffering.*
**—Dalai Lama**

In order for the *Says Who?* method to work, you have to be willing to **"work the method,"** and, by that I mean, be ready to face your negative thoughts by really listening to them in your mind as you're thinking them, no matter how unappealing, embarrassing, or frightening they may be. You have to be willing to say to yourself, "Bring it on! I'm ready to face my powerful mind, and all it has to reveal to me." Once you're ready to do that, you can go ahead and question, confront, challenge, and ultimately change any thought that does not serve your well-being.

Everyone has the ability to change their negative thoughts and beliefs about themselves if they really want to. They just have to commit to doing it as a **daily discipline**, like brushing your teeth. I use brushing your teeth as an analogy because that's something we know we have to do daily in order to maintain the health of our teeth and gums, so it's automatic for us. That's exactly what I'm recommending for a healthy mind: the same daily discipline you would give to the physical parts of yourself that you need to take care of and manage properly.

*Says Who?* is that daily discipline. As I said in Chapter One, we can think up to 70,000 thoughts per day, and some of those are bound to be negative. So if we can get ourselves in the habit of questioning those daily negative thoughts once they crop up instead of letting them go unchallenged, we can make a difference in how our thoughts work. If you don't make the commitment to change your negative thoughts and beliefs about yourself by questioning them with the *Says Who?* method with consistency, you run the risk of getting right back on that negative hamster wheel of thinking, and your mind starts to recycle the same negative thoughts that have been playing over and over again in your mind before. Those thoughts will stick around as long as you let them, and the way you allow for that is by not questioning them with the *Says Who?* method to find out what they're doing in your mind. They're not going anywhere until you let them go, hence, question 7: "Do I want to keep this thought or let it go?" Let it go!

As I mentioned earlier, you can't change your negative thoughts by questioning them "some of the time", and letting them slide other times. The *Says Who?* method isn't something you do Monday, Wednesday, and Friday, and let your mind be up to its old clever tricks the rest of the days of the week.

Changing the way we think takes practice. It takes a **daily discipline**. As much as I'd like to say that just "thinking positive" is going to do the trick, I can't because it *won't*. Yes, thinking positive thoughts will put you on the right thinking track, but it's **"staying positive"** that matters even more, and that's what the *Says Who?* method does: it keeps your thoughts positive and productive consistently so they can serve your well being, not disrupt it. It's too easy to fall into a negative place about yourself as soon as an obstacle pops up, like problems at work or in a relationship, or even succumbing to temptation by having that cigarette, drink, or snack you want to avoid. Life is full of those unexpected obstacles! But if you are practiced at questioning your thoughts, you will be better equipped at handling life's problems and challenges in a productive, proactive way and be better able to handle the obstacles when they do arise.

The *Says Who?* method is intended for you to use to support your innermost desires, and help you reach your goals by challenging any negative thought that is trying to undermine or defeat you to achieve what you want. Think of it as a way to filter out or eliminate any thought that does not support you 100%. Who doesn't need a support system to help keep us motivated and believing in ourselves? Sometimes you can't rely on a friend or family member to be that motivator or cheerleader for you—you've got to rely on yourself. *Says Who?* will give you strength to face and confront your own inner obstacles or resistance to change. At the end of the day, we have to face who we really are on our own because no one can fight our "true identity" battles for us.

If there's one thing we all have in common, it's that we need a practice or discipline to keep us on the straight and narrow, and accepting and loving of ourselves. For some, it could be meditation or yoga that keeps them connected to their center or core being, and for others who are concerned about keeping their weight under control and being healthy, they might have an exercise routine they feel works for them. Whatever it is we want to achieve, realize or accomplish in our lives, **the name of the game is consistency**, and that's exactly what the *Says Who?* method will help you with—being consistent about keeping your thoughts positive and productive so that you can realize your desires and achieve your goals, whatever they may be. The sky's the limit!

However, the method is not something you can do just once and expect it to change the way you think. It takes practice and it needs to be incorporated into your daily routine in order to be truly effective. With time and practice this will become second nature for you and you won't tolerate old negative beliefs to affect or influence your current positive thoughts because you'll know that your thoughts ultimately dictate your beliefs, which affects your behavior and how you feel. The point is success is achieved by making the process a daily habit. You need to adhere to a discipline—it's too easy to get lazy, distracted or give into temptation. Luckily, the *Says Who?* method is simple and easy to adopt, and can be done anywhere and anytime. It's hard to make excuses not to do it because the truth is, how difficult is it to ask yourself the first question, Says who?, which takes a second, and just by doing that alone, even if you asked yourself nothing else, you're already sending a message to your mind that you're in charge of your thinking by deciding what thoughts you want to let in and which ones you don't.

I want to emphasize that **the work must be done, by you, for you,** and in order for you to change the negativity you believe or think about yourself, you must question it, challenge it, and transform it. Everyone can change an old negative thought or belief they hold about themselves into a positive one, and by doing so, can then change their thoughts to support a healthier, "accurate" perception of themselves if they make a commitment to do so.

Remember, you are what you think, and what you think creates your reality. By using the *Says Who?* method, you can transform your thinking to be exactly what you want it to be to manifest the life you desire and deserve.

## Chapter 18
# Working the *Says Who?* Method

*The three great essentials to achieve anything worthwhile are:*
*hard work, stick-to-itiveness, and common sense.*
**—Thomas A. Edison**

W hen you become more practiced with the *Says Who?* method, you will find that whenever a negative or fear-based thought pops up in your mind, you'll be quick to ask yourself any of the questions, and they will redirect your thoughts right back on a positive track.

However, as I emphasized in the last chapter, the key to becoming more proficient at the method so that it becomes second nature and most effective is by making it a daily practice. Incorporate it into your routine, making it an important discipline or ritual, like exercise. Taking a few minutes each day to "check in" with yourself will help orient you and keep you on a positive track.

Remember—it's one thing to think a positive thought, but it's a lot more challenging to *keep* your thoughts that way, because we have so many thoughts coming in and out of our minds daily. That's why it's important to not only be hyper aware of them, but also vigilant in keeping them productive and constructive, which you can do by using the *Says Who?* method. That way, when you're confronted with a situation that brings up fear, worry or self-doubt—and no matter how good you may feel about yourself on any given day, insecurity, anxiety or critical thoughts are bound to pop up: your boss demeans you, your spouse or partner hurts your feelings, you experience a loss, or some kind of frustration—you will be better prepared to question your feelings and reactions, and how best to respond to them.

Think of it like running a marathon. Anyone can do it if they want to badly enough. However, we all know you don't just go out the first day, strap on your Nikes and run 26 miles. It's an incremental thing. The minute you start running, your mind can easily say, "I can't do this! I can't run this far!" *Or* you can tell yourself that you will start small and improve a little every day, which is a positive thought that supports your desire. That way when you do finally run the big race you're prepared.

That can apply to anything you do that is challenging or pushing you beyond your comfort zone. When people train themselves for something that requires physical stamina, they not only have to build their body strength, but they need to increase their mind strength. One cannot work without the other. Everything begins with a single thought that inspires you into action. Our thoughts literally power the engine that takes us where we want to go.

The *Says Who?* method helps you be in the best mental shape you can, and strengthen your mind power to approach whatever it is you want to do or accomplish. Like an athlete who trains daily, you need to train your mind consistently to stay focused on fulfilling your desires and realizing your goals.

If you don't have day-in/day-out discipline, which is what this method is about, that is, the questions that lead you to thoughts that support your desires and goals, it's too easy to fall back into that negative place once again. We all need a daily practice to keep our thoughts wholesome and positive to make sure they don't stray into negativity, frustration and self-defeat.

I want you to think of your mind as a muscle you can strengthen a little more each day. And just like any muscle in your body can become weak and flaccid when you don't use it, so can your mind strength. And it's not like you have to do anything arduous, like going to the gym to keep your body strong. You simply need to be aware of your negative thoughts, and manage them properly so they don't disrupt your well-being. That's not very demanding, is it?

When you become very familiar with the *Says Who?* method, the questions will be like having your own personal trainer in your mind that can whip a negative thought into shape faster than you can imagine! Let the method work for you, but you first have to be willing to **work the method!**

We all know how easy it is to get lazy and complacent, especially when things are going well and the negative thoughts have receded. However, we are wise enough to know, and experience has taught us, that negative thoughts or feelings can pop up unannounced at almost any time, particularly when an unexpected stressful incident arrives— loss of a job, a sudden change in a relationship, an illness—on our doorstep. Even the stressful events that are not surprises, such as a child going off to college, an impending marriage or divorce, or changing careers, can also trigger negativity or fear.

Those are the times when we are quick to go into *reactive mode*.

What I want you to get familiar with and good at is being able to shift gears quickly into *observer mode* so you can ask yourself any of the seven *Says Who?* questions to help calm you down and ground you. I know that you might not always be able to immediately ask yourself the questions when something has gotten you down, worried or upset, but if you find that you are really plugged into something that's happened, and it's making things worse for you, try to at least ask yourself one of the questions like, "Does this thought make me feel better?" or "Am I in control of this thought?" If you answer with a definitive "No!" then acknowledge that your negative thought is causing you more distress or anxiety by saying to yourself, "This thought is making me feel worse so I'm going to let it go." You may also find that just repeating the words "Let it go," is also effective, and can be used whenever you need a simple mantra for releasing a thought.

Repeating any of the seven *Says Who?* questions over and over again to yourself will help it stay in the foreground of your mind. If you're someone who likes to meditate (and even if you're not, you can still try this), you can sit somewhere quiet, close your eyes, take a few deep breaths in and out, and repeat any of these questions:

1. *Says who?*
2. *Have I heard someone say this thought before?*
3. *Do I like this thought?*
4. *Does this thought make me feel better?*
5. *Does this thought work for me?*
6. *Am I in control of this thought?*
7. *Do I want to keep this thought or let it go?*

You will find that by putting your focus on any of these questions, something might come up for you that could be helpful or useful for what you need to know. It could be the answer you're looking for beyond just "yes" or "no"—maybe something deeper that has personal meaning for you, and gives you a better understanding about yourself. Sitting quietly with ourselves can help us get to the core of what we need to. It's like finding that missing piece of the puzzle we're looking for, and these seven questions can help you find it.

The *Says Who?* method will help you stay centered and focused, providing a discipline and structure to ensure that you are constantly keeping your thoughts in check—to make sure you are in control of them, not them of you. However, making this a daily practice can often be easier said than done. That's why I've devised a Workbook to help you get started and develop your positive thought muscle. Think of it as your "mental gym" where you can literally "lift" your thoughts up! And there's something about seeing your progress written down on paper that mirrors back to you that you're on the right track.

The Workbook is designed to be customized to each person, and the responses to the questions and exercises are intended to elicit answers that will allow you to better understand the origin and purpose of your thoughts, and steer them in the direction that serves who you are, and what you want to do in the best way possible. The great thing about our thoughts is that they change. They don't have to stay fixed or permanent. We can be creative with them, which is exciting. Imagine that you've got this incredible mind that is full of endless possibilities, as far as what you can fill it with, and here is your opportunity to do that. As much as I want you to take this process seriously, I still want you to have fun with it, and by doing that, I mean, don't criticize yourself in the process!

Asking yourself the first question—"Says who?"—will set the tone for you to begin exploring your mind, and get to know any thought better that has (or needs) your attention. There's something empowering about being able to answer the question "Says who?" with "Says me," because that means that you are taking responsibility for having a thought that needs to be confronted and challenged, and you're ready to do that. You're not pushing your thought aside, or denying having it, and even if it's a thought that causes you unhappiness or fear, you are ready to "own it", and deal with it.

With practice, you will get skillful and swift at using the *Says Who?* questions to your advantage and able to change or stop a negative or fear-based thought with ease. I find myself using question 6: "Does this thought work for me?" whenever a thought comes up that begins to take me out of the present moment. If I don't feel that my thought is working for me favorably, and I sense that it's stirring up something that doesn't feel real or authentic, I use it immediately. Another one of my favorites is question 4: "Does this thought make me feel better?" which helps me know almost immediately if it does or doesn't. You might find yourself using some questions more than others, or perhaps different ones at different times, or you might feel more comfortable using them all, but whatever ones you do use, make sure to use them with frequency and consistency so that a discipline is developed to keep your thoughts present and conscious.

The *Says Who?* Workbook is your own personal journal that you *create*, which is designed to help you accomplish two things:

- First—help you know your negative thoughts better by identifying them.
- Second—help you transform your negative thoughts into positive ones by changing them.

Use this workbook like a diary. Daily entries are helpful to gauge what's on your mind and also get you into the habit of acknowledging your thoughts as a daily practice. You can jot down any thoughts you're having, have had, can't stop having, or want to let go of having. This will help you get more familiar with your thoughts so you can manage them better. What you write down, is not meant to be judged or criticized in any way because it would be counterproductive to what you're trying to work through and change. Write down whatever you want, even if it's uncomfortable, embarrassing, or painful. The more honest, revealing, and daring you can be, the better. This is your opportunity to get as real with yourself as you can!

**Get ready to own, change, and love your thoughts!**

## Chapter 19

# The Workbook

To begin the *Says who?* method, it's important to remember these three things when you have a thought you want to work on:

1. Acknowledge it
2. Observe it
3. Do not react to it

Your thoughts will be broken down into these categories:

1. Negative
2. Fear-based
3. Judgmental
4. Worried

You will write them in a "Thought Chart" which is divided into three segments:

1. **Question**—where you will *inquire* about your thoughts;
2. **Examination**—where you will *investigate* your thoughts;
3. **Realization**—where you will *discover* the origin and purpose of your thoughts.

Below, make a list of your negative, fear-based, judgmental or worried thoughts, which occur most frequently:

**NEGATIVE THOUGHTS:**
**EXAMPLE:** *"I feel like a failure."*

| |
|---|
| 1. |
| 2. |
| 3. |
| 4. |
| 5. |

Now, incorporate any one of them into the following chart to help you work the *Says Who?* method. For instance, say that one of the negative thoughts you wrote down is, "I feel like a failure."

| THOUGHT CHART: "I feel like a failure." | | |
|---|---|---|
| **Question** | **Examination** | **Realization** |
| Says Who? | Who says I'm a failure? | My mother used to compare me to my sister when I was growing up and that made me feel like I was a failure. |
| Have I heard someone say this thought before? | Is that my own thought or did I hear someone tell me I'm a failure before? | Sometimes I can hear my mother's voice in my head, comparing me to my sister, and it sounds like she's calling me a failure. |
| Do I like this thought? | Do I like thinking that I'm a failure? | I don't like thinking I'm a failure. When that happens, I feel hopeless and powerless to do anything about it. |
| Does this thought make me feel better? | Does thinking I'm a failure make me feel better about myself? | Thinking I'm a failure makes me feel really bad about myself like I'm never going to be good enough. |
| Does this thought work for me? | Does thinking I'm a failure work for me in a positive or productive way, or add anything to my life? | Thinking I'm a failure does nothing positive for me other than make me feel bad and insecure. |

| Am I in control of this thought? | Do I feel like I can control or manage this thought that I'm a failure when it comes up for me? | I don't feel like I'm in control of thinking I'm a failure when it comes up, but I'd like to have power over that thought. |
|---|---|---|
| Do I want to keep this thought or let it go? | Do I want to hold onto the thought that I'm a failure or do I want to get rid of it by letting it go? | I don't want to keep thinking that I'm a failure and I absolutely want to let that negative thought go! |

Now, create your own **THOUGHT CHART** below, making one chart for each negative thought:

| THOUGHT CHART: | | |
|---|---|---|
| **Question** | **Examination** | **Realization** |
| Says Who? | | |
| Have I heard someone say this thought before? | | |
| Do I like this thought? | | |
| Does this thought make me feel better? | | |
| Does this thought work for me? | | |

| | | |
|---|---|---|
| Am I in control of this thought? | | |
| Do I want to keep this thought or let it go? | | |

Repeat this by writing down your Fear-Based thought, then answering the *Says Who?* questions in the Thought Chart:

**FEAR-BASED THOUGHTS:**
**EXAMPLE**: *"I'm afraid I'm going to end up alone."*

| | |
|---|---|
| 1. | |
| 2. | |
| 3. | |
| 4. | |
| 5. | |

| THOUGHT CHART: | | |
|---|---|---|
| **Question** | **Examination** | **Realization** |
| Says Who? | | |
| Have I heard someone say this thought before? | | |
| Do I like this thought? | | |
| Does this thought make me feel better? | | |

| | | |
|---|---|---|
| Does this thought work for me? | | |
| Am I in control of this thought? | | |
| Do I want to keep this thought or let it go? | | |

## JUDGMENTAL THOUGHTS:

**EXAMPLE**: *"People who are well educated are smarter than me."*

| | |
|---|---|
| 1. | |
| 2. | |
| 3. | |
| 4. | |
| 5. | |

| THOUGHT CHART: | | |
|---|---|---|
| **Question** | **Examination** | **Realization** |
| Says Who? | | I |
| Have I heard someone say this thought before? | | |
| Do I like this thought? | | |
| Does this thought make me feel better? | | |
| Does this thought work for me? | | |

| | | |
|---|---|---|
| Am I in control of this thought? | | |
| Do I want to keep this thought or let it go? | | |

**WORRIED THOUGHTS:**

**EXAMPLE:** *"I'm not going to make enough money."*

| |
|---|
| 1. |
| 2. |
| 3. |
| 4. |
| 5. |

| THOUGHT CHART: | | |
|---|---|---|
| **Question** | **Examination** | **Realization** |
| Says Who? | | |
| Have I heard someone say this thought before? | | |
| Do I like this thought? | | |
| Does this thought make me feel better? | | |
| Does this thought work for me? | | |
| Am I in control of this thought? | | |

| Do I want to keep this thought or let it go? | | |
|---|---|---|
| | | |

## DESIRES AND GOALS:

Just as it's important to identify your negative, fear-based, judgmental, and worried thoughts, it's equally essential to declare your desires and goals. By writing them down, you can see the distinct difference between them—your negative type thoughts being "unproductive," and your desires and goals being "productive." When a negative thought is coupled with a positive desire or goal, it will cancel it out because it cannot support what is trying to be attained or achieved. Only positive thoughts can carry a desire or goal into action.

**Make a list of your Desires & Goals:**
**DESIRES:**
**EXAMPLE:** *"I want a better job."*

| 1. |
|---|
| 2. |
| 3. |
| 4. |
| 5. |

**GOALS:**
**EXAMPLE:** *"I'm going to get the job I want by six months."*

| 1. |
|---|
| 2. |
| 3. |
| 4. |
| 5. |

Now, take the thoughts you wrote down in any of the categories—Negative, Fearful, Judgmental, Worried—and combine them with any of your Desires or Goals. This creates a **CONFLICTING SENTENCE**, which is a thought that does not match or support your desire or goal.

**FEARFUL THOUGHT:**
**EXAMPLE**: *"I'm afraid I'm unqualified to get the job I want."*

**DESIRE/GOAL:**
**EXAMPLE:** *"I would love to get a job as an editor of a popular magazine."*

**CONFLICTING SENTENCE:**
**EXAMPLE** *"I would love to get a job as an editor of a popular magazine, but I'm unqualified to get a job like that."*

**CONFLICTING SENTENCES:**

| | |
|---|---|
| 1. | |
| 2. | |
| 3. | |
| 4. | |
| 5. | |

## CHANGE A CONFLICTING SENTENCE TO A NON-CONFLICTING SENTENCE:

Now, take your Negative, Fearful, Judgmental, or Worried thoughts, and change them to match and support your Desire/Goal.

**EXAMPLE:** *"I would love to get a job as an editor of a popular magazine, and feel like I could bring a lot to it."*

Now, continue changing your Negative, Fearful, Judgmental, or Worried thoughts to positive ones, and combine them with your Desire/Goal.

**NON-CONFLICTING SENTENCES:**

| |
|---|
| 1. |
| 2. |
| 3. |
| 4. |
| 5. |

**RELEASE & REPLACE:**

Now that you've changed your **CONFLICTING THOUGHT** to a **NON-CONFLICTING THOUGHT**, you've **RELEASED** a negative or fearful thought that was opposing your desire or goal, and **REPLACED** it with a positive and productive thought that can support your **DESIRE/GOAL.**

Make a list of the thoughts you **RELEASED**, followed by the thoughts you **REPLACED** them with.

**RELEASED:**

**EXAMPLE:** *"I'm unqualified to get the job I want."*

| |
|---|
| 1. |
| 2. |
| 3. |
| 4. |
| 5. |

**REPLACED:**
**EXAMPLE:** *"I feel like I could bring a lot to it."*

| |
|---|
| 1. |
| 2. |
| 3. |
| 4. |
| 5. |

When you hold Non-Conflicting Sentences in your mind, they can support your Desire/Goal, which then means you are ready to create your **ACTION THOUGHTS**. Those are the positive thoughts that tell your subconscious what you want to do proactively, and propel you towards your desires and goals. Here's how you take a Non-Conflicting Sentence and make it an Action Thought:

**NON-CONFLICTING SENTENCE:**
**EXAMPLE**: *"I would love to get a job as an editor of a popular magazine, and feel like I could bring a lot to it."*

**ACTION THOUGHT:**
**EXAMPLE:** *"I'm going to send my resume out this week to three popular magazine publishers."*

You can see how your Non-Conflicting sentence lends itself to an Action Thought for you to go after your goal. When your thoughts are positive, clear and definitive, you can go after what you want.

Make a list of your Action Thoughts -- the things you want to do or go after.

**ACTION THOUGHTS:**

| |
|---|
| 1. |
| 2. |
| 3. |
| 4. |
| 5. |

Now that you've made your list of **ACTION THOUGHTS**, keep track of them by writing them down on a calendar. This will help you get even more specific and pro-active with your desires and goals by putting them down on the months and days you want to move forward with them. However, if you don't act on your action thoughts on the date you've written down, be very careful that you don't slip back into allowing for negative, critical or judgmental thoughts. And if you do, go back and write them down again in the negative thought column in your workbook, and work the *Says Who?* method on them.

This workbook is intended to be used in whatever area you need working on. Just because you find yourself in an **ACTION THOUGHT** phase, does not mean you've eradicated negative thinking. Remember, negative thoughts will come and go in your mind at different times. The *Says Who?* method is about learning how to manage them better.

**ACTION THOUGHTS ACTED ON:**

It's great turning negative thoughts into **NON-CONFLICTING SENTENCES**, and then into **ACTION THOUGHTS,** but it's even better when you've actually acted on them. Make a list of the **ACTION THOUGHTS** you've put into action by doing them.

**EXAMPLE:** *"I emailed my resume to a few popular magazines."*

| |
|---|
| 1. |
| 2. |
| 3. |
| 4. |
| 5. |

**POSITIVE AFFIRMATIONS:**

It feels really good when we follow through on our **ACTION THOUGHTS,** and a good way to support our efforts is to follow up with positive affirmations.

**EXAMPLE:** *"I am confident about getting a job, and will not give up until I get one."*

Make a list of **POSITIVE AFFIRMATIONS** that support your **ACTION THOUGHTS** you've **ACTED ON:**

| |
|---|
| 1. |
| 2. |
| 3. |
| 4. |
| 5. |

**ACTION RESULTS:**

Acting on your **ACTION THOUGHTS** is necessary in changing negative thought patterns. By doing it with consistency you're building the mind strength needed to not slip into old mental patterns of laziness or complacency. When you've proven to yourself that you can "walk your thought," by acting on it, you're programming your mind to not only think positive, but to remain positive. It replaces "I can't" with "I did," and once you've acted on what your desire is to reach your goal, it's hard to go back to "Non-Action" thinking. By supporting your efforts with **POSITIVE AFFIRMATIONS**, you're acknowledging what you're doing, which is important to do for recognizing how far you've come in transforming your thinking. Getting results out of putting your **ACTION THOUGHTS** into motion is what you hope to accomplish, but keep in mind that sometimes the results we get aren't always exactly what we had hoped for, or in the exact time frame we'd like.

Remember, we think positive thoughts first and foremost because it makes us feel good about ourselves and serves our well-being. If the outcome of our efforts is what we wanted, that's great, but if not, there's still something positive to gain by simply putting ourselves out there and not being afraid to do so. Whatever the results are of your efforts, write down what you got out of ACTING ON your **ACTION THOUGHTS**.

**EXAMPLE:** *"I overcame my fear and insecurity by applying for a job where the competition is really fierce."*

| | |
|---|---|
| 1. | |
| 2. | |
| 3. | |
| 4. | |
| 5. | |

**CHANGING NEGATIVE BELIEFS TO POSITIVE ONES:**

Our negative beliefs stay stored in our subconscious until we change them. Unlike a negative thought that can come and go, a negative belief is usually fixed, and will stay that way until we change it. Writing down your negative beliefs will let you see what you're holding onto. Questioning them with the *Says Who?* method will help you find out if it's your original thought, or someone else's that you took on as your own, and if you're ready to let them go.

**EXAMPLE:** *"I have to please others before myself because I'm less deserving."*

This type of belief would influence how someone views themselves, and what they feel they're worthy of. The decisions they make in their life can also be affected by this belief in some way.

Write down your **NEGATIVE BELIEFS**:

| |
|---|
| 1. |
| 2. |
| 3. |
| 4. |
| 5. |

**Work your negative beliefs in the Thought Chart:**

| Thought Chart | | |
|---|---|---|
| **Question** | **Examination** | **Realization** |
| Says Who? | | |
| Have I heard someone say this thought before? | | |
| Do I like this thought? | | |
| Does this thought make me feel better? | | |
| Does this thought work for me? | | |

| Am I in control of this thought? | | |
|---|---|---|
| Do I want to keep this thought or let it go? | | |

## POSITIVE BELIEFS

Write down your **CHANGED BELIEFS**:

**EXAMPLE:** *"I am deserving of pleasing myself as much as anyone else."*

| 1. |
|---|
| 2. |
| 3. |
| 4. |
| 5. |

## SERVING YOUR WELL-BEING:

The *Says Who?* method is intended to keep your thoughts positive and productive to support your **DESIRES/GOALS**, and to serve your **WELL-BEING**, which is a state of being happy and healthy. It's important for us to know and recognize the things that contribute to our **WELL-BEING**, and go towards them in our life.

Make a list of thoughts that **SERVE YOUR WELL-BEING**, and support you being happy and healthy—mind, body and spirit.

**EXAMPLE**: *"I feel happy when I'm with people I can completely be myself with."*

| | |
|---|---|
| 1. | |
| 2. | |
| 3. | |
| 4. | |
| 5. | |

**NOT SERVING YOUR WELL-BEING:**
Make a list of thoughts that don't serve your well-being:
**EXAMPLE:** *"I can't stand up for myself."*

| | |
|---|---|
| 1. | |
| 2. | |
| 3. | |
| 4. | |
| 5. | |

**Identifying the thoughts that serve your well-being, and thoughts that don't, helps you know which ones to question that need to be changed.**

Use the **Thought Chart** for thoughts that don't serve your well-being:

THOUGHT CHART

| Question | Examination | Realization |
|---|---|---|
| Says who? | | |
| Do I like this thought? | | |

| | | |
|---|---|---|
| Does this thought make me feel better? | | |
| Does this thought work for me? | | |
| Am I in control of this thought? | | |
| Do I want to keep this thought or let it go? | | |

**PUTTING YOUR WELL-BEING THOUGHTS INTO ACTION:**

Now that you've written down the thoughts that support your well-being, and the ones that don't, write down the ones that do in an action sentence.

**EXAMPLE:** *"I will spend more time with people that I can be completely myself with."*

| |
|---|
| 1. |
| 2. |
| 3. |
| 4. |
| 5. |

**DECLARING WHO I AM:**

Deciding what you want your thoughts to be is taking charge of your life, and what you want to manifest for yourself. It's like you're declaring your authentic self to the universe. Write down who you are today, which is different than who you've been at any other time in your life.

**EXAMPLE:** *"I feel more creative than I ever have before, and I'm unafraid to express it."*

| | |
|---|---|
| 1. | |
| 2. | |
| 3. | |
| 4. | |
| 5. | |

**VISUALIZING WHO I AM:**

Now that you've declared who you are to the universe, visualize what that looks like. It can be how you see yourself, and where you see yourself. And just like the delicious apple we envision biting into is juicy, red, or green, you too are just as desirable!

**EXAMPLE:** *"I see myself traveling to places I've never been to before and having wonderful new experiences. I'm happy and content. My life is good!"*

| | |
|---|---|
| 1. | |
| 2. | |
| 3. | |
| 4. | |
| 5. | |

**A THOUGHT CHECK-UP:**

In addition to the Workbook, sometimes it's helpful to do a periodic thought "check-up" as a way to stay on top of and monitor the types of thoughts you have. It's another tool to help track whether negative thoughts are threatening to dominate or overtake your state of mind and question them before they do. That's why I devised a short Questionnaire to help lead you through the process. You might like recording your answers in a journal because the process of writing things down can help clarify your thoughts and show "thinking patterns," which is what can happen when your thoughts go unquestioned and are left to become repetitive or intensified. Either way, it's a valuable supplement to the *Says Who?* method as a way to perform a reality check on your thoughts:

## A Questionaire About Your Thoughts:

During the day are your thoughts mostly (Circle your answers):

- Positive or negative?
- Ruled by fear, worry/doubt, or by confidence?
- In the present, past or future?
- Supportive of your desires or goals?
- Self-critical or critical of others, or both?
- Judgmental of yourself or of others, or both?
- Self-loving or loving of others, or both?
- Empowering or undermining?
- Guilt-ridden or shameful?
- Happy or sad?
- Optimistic or pessimistic?
- Nice?
- Mindful?
- Practical?
- Realistic?
- Creative?
- Spiritual?
- Visionary?
- Original?
- Funny?
- Serious?
- Delusional

- Odd?
- Narcissistic?
- Harmful?
- Violent?
- Repetitive?
- Predictable?
- Surprising?
- Serve your well-being?

And finally, are you pleased with most of your thoughts?
Yes / No

## A Thought Game:

You've done quite a bit of work on getting to know your thoughts better by being honest with yourself, which isn't always easy to do, so I'd like to balance it with something still related to getting to know your thoughts—but fun! This is a lighthearted game to play with yourself or other people. Ask the following questions, and answer them with the very first word that pops up in your mind. Don't hesitate or censor your answers. Also, try not to judge or criticize yours or someone else's answers, but if you do, ask yourself the *Says Who?* questions to find out why you are being critical or judgmental. This is just another way to find out how we think:

| |
|---|
| Walking on the beach makes me feel |
| Dancing makes me feel |
| Eating makes me feel |
| Making love makes me feel |
| Laughing makes me feel |
| Getting attention makes me feel |
| Getting compliments makes me feel |

| |
|---|
| Getting criticized makes me feel |
| Getting affection makes me feel |
| Having love in my life makes me feel |
| Not having love in my life makes me feel |
| Making money makes me feel |
| Not having money makes me feel |
| Asking for what I want makes me feel |
| Getting what I want makes me feel |
| Not getting what I want makes me feel |
| Getting hurt makes me feel |
| Getting acknowledgment makes me feel |
| Not getting acknowledgment makes me feel |
| Being around people I love makes me feel |
| Being around strangers makes me feel |
| Being around men makes me feel |
| Being around women makes me feel |
| Being around animals makes me feel |
| Being around elderly people makes me feel |
| Being around children makes me feel |
| Being disrespected makes me feel |
| Being respected makes me feel |
| Working makes me feel |
| Not working makes me feel |
| Doing the things I love makes me feel |
| Doing the things I don't love makes me feel |
| Being honest makes me feel |
| Being dishonest makes me feel |
| Being in control makes me feel |
| Letting go of control makes me feel |
| Thinking about my childhood makes me feel |
| Thinking about getting older makes me feel |

| |
|---|
| Being quiet makes me feel |
| Taking time for myself makes me feel |
| Being spiritual makes me feel |
| Thinking about death makes me feel |
| Thinking about fulfilling my purpose makes me feel |
| Being seen for who I really am makes me feel |

*Did you find your answers were (check as many as apply):*

- Surprising
- Not surprising
- Predictable
- Enlightening
- Uncomfortable
- Comfortable
- Funny

You can play this game over and over again, and if you really do say the very first word that pops in your mind, it may very well be different than the last time you asked yourself or someone else these questions. Remember, thoughts come and go. We're the ones that hold on to them. You can also make up your own questions too, which keeps it interesting.

## And Finally—A Thought For The Day:
You might have a book or calendar of inspiring thoughts or quotes you like. How about creating your own—with your thoughts! You can start your day with one of your motivating thoughts that makes you feel good, or end the day with a soothing one when you're lying in bed before you go to sleep. Maybe it's a thought of gratitude, or love. Whatever it is, it's nice to be able to jot it down, and refer to it

at another time. You don't have to be a poet to write a little "gem" or "pearl" that resonates for you. Give it a try and see what you come up with:

| MONDAY |
|---|
| TUESDAY |
| WEDNESDAY |
| THURSDAY |
| FRIDAY |
| SATURDAY |
| SUNDAY |

## Snapshot: Recapping The *Says Who?* Method & Workbook:

### *The Method:*

1. Acknowledge a negative thought
2. Be the observer
3. Not the reactor
4. Ask yourself the 7 *Says Who?* questions:
   - Says who?
   - Have I heard someone say this thought before?
   - Do I like this thought?
   - Does this thought make me feel better?
   - Does this thought work for me?
   - Am I in control of this thought?
   - Do I want to keep this thought or let it go?

### *Workbook:*

Use this list to check off, in order, what work you need to do, or have done, to realize your WELL-BEING:

1. Identify:
   - Negative Thoughts
   - Fearful Thoughts
   - Judgmental Thoughts
   - Worried Thoughts
2. Apply 7 *Says Who?* questions to thoughts
3. Identify:
   - Desires
   - Goals
   - Conflicting Thoughts
   - Non-Conflicting Thoughts
4. Release your Negative Thoughts and Replace with Positive Thoughts
5. Identify Action Thoughts
6. Use Action Thought Calendar
7. Identify Action Thoughts Acted On
8. Positive Affirmations
9. Action Results
10. Changing Negative Beliefs
11. Apply 7 *Says Who?* Questions
12. Identify Changed Beliefs
    - Serving Your Well-Being
    - Putting Well-Being into Action
    - Declaring Who I am
    - Visualizing Who I am
    - A Thought For The Day

## Chapter 20

# Mindfulness Meditation: Taking A Break From Thinking

*To understand the immeasurable,*
*the mind must be extraordinarily quiet, still.*
—**Jiddu Krishnamurti**

Getting to know our thoughts better by questioning them with the *Says Who?* method is a great way to find out what occupies our minds, and if our thoughts are serving our well-being. By recognizing thoughts that don't nurture or replenish us, we can eliminate them from our mind by "transforming" them into ones that do.

But sometimes during the day, it's equally important to stop the activity and chatter in our minds (even if it's positive chatter) by simply giving it a well-deserved break, and there's no better way to do that than to meditate. Dedicating ten to twenty minutes (twice a day if you can) to sitting quietly and being in the present with total awareness, will help quiet and calm your mind, and make you feel more relaxed and peaceful. I suggest doing the following Mindfulness Meditation when you're not using the *Says Who?* method or the workbook. There's a time to be with our thoughts—confront them, investigate them, and challenge them, and then there's a time to let them just "be."

## Mindfulness Meditation:

Mindfulness Meditation is about being in the present moment with total awareness and non-judgment. Simply be aware, and "mindful" of whatever happens, and try not to stop yourself from thinking. During your meditation be aware of what your thoughts are, and anything your senses might be experiencing. Try not to analyze or judge your thoughts or feelings, but just allow them to "be."

Sit on a chair with your legs uncrossed and feet on the ground, or a meditation cushion either cross-legged or extended straight out. It's important that wherever you sit it's comfortable for you, and if you need support for your back sit somewhere that can do that.

Place your hands on your lap. You can put them either palm-down on your thighs, cup your left hand over your right, or palms up with your thumb and first finger touching.

Close your eyes, and try to relax the muscles around them. Take a deep breath in and a deep breath out. Continue to put your focus on your breath, and simply notice it flowing in, and flowing out. Don't force or manipulate your breathing, just allow yourself to breathe as naturally as you can.

As you breathe in, silently say the word "In," and as you exhale, say the word "Out." You can also say "Rising" and "Falling away" or "Letting go." If you find that your mind is becoming active, gently bring your focus back to your breath. Repeat this throughout your meditation.

Bring your awareness back to ending your meditation. Rub your palms together and place them over your eyes and face, or your heart, feeling the warmth coming from your hands. Put your hands down and open your eyes. Take the time you need to gently transition to whatever you're going to do next in your day.

Taking the time to quiet your mind with Mindfulness Meditation is caring for yourself in the same way you "mindfully" pay attention to the thoughts you think each day with the *Says Who?* method. These two practices together are wonderful disciplines for becoming more thoughtful, compassionate, and conscious.

# Chapter 21
## *Says Who?* Says You!

*You have power over your mind—not outside events.*
*Realize this, and you will find strength.*

**—Marcus Aurelius**

Now that you understand how the *Says Who?* Method works, and realize that you are the creator of your thoughts, are you ready to let them serve your well-being in the best way possible?

Each day you wake up, you can declare to the universe exactly what you want to manifest. You hold the key to the doorway of your mind. Are you ready to walk through it, and let each thought be a step towards living your dreams?

Imagine what incredible ideas you can conjure up in your mind, which is as boundless as the sea. Let what you envision be bold and fearless. Go after what your mind dares you to think. You are the master of your internal dialogue, the commander of the ship that is sailing towards your destiny, but you must navigate your thoughts carefully so they can guide you on your journey, and help you get to your desired destination with clarity and authenticity.

Let the "*Says Who?*" method be your map, and when the waters get choppy, you will know exactly how to keep yourself afloat by asking yourself the seven questions that hold your thoughts accountable, and keep them honest and real. Now is the time to know your mind better than you ever have before, and if you are truly ready to set sail towards your destiny, begin today with thoughts that tell you that you are a champion, a leader, a visionary, and that there is nothing you cannot do.

Face your thoughts daily, each and every one of them. Ask them what they want you to know, and if any of your thoughts tell you something other than "You can do whatever you put your mind to", question and challenge them by asking, "*Says Who?*" Only then can you realize that it is you that holds the answer you are seeking, and that answer is "Says me!"

You are the ruler of your mind, and your thoughts serve you. Let them be your dutiful soldiers. Tell them what you want them to do for you, where you want them to go, and what you need from them to thrive and succeed. Make sure they support and praise you, and tell you that you are worthy and lovable, and if they tell you otherwise, let your thoughts know that you create them, and as fast as they are born, is as quick as you can remove them from your mind as if they never existed.

You are the true master of your mind. Design your thoughts to be your greatest invention, paint them to be your most exquisite masterpiece, conduct them to be a brilliant symphony of words.

# About The Author

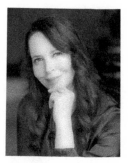

**Ora Nadrich** is a certified Life Coach, and Mindfulness Meditation teacher. She is a frequent blogger for the Huffington Post on Mindfulness, and leads workshops on "Living a Mindful Life."

Ora was an actress and screenwriter, where she worked in film, episodic television, and commercials for more than a decade, which she feels provided her vast experience in exploring motivation and the process of self-discovery. During that time, she simultaneously embarked on a two-decade psychological and spiritual journey towards self-awareness and transformation.

Ora retired from acting, and devoted her time to studying the workings of the mind. On her psychological and spiritual journey she explored Cognitive Behavioral Therapy (CBT), and a multi-year, intensive study of various disciplines and techniques, including the Technology of Change with Robert Lorenz, and extensive Jungian analysis. She studied Kabbalah and Buddhism, and met some of the finest spiritual teachers and leaders like, Gurumayi of Siddha Yoga, Sonam Kazi, the Dalai Lama's interpreter, and, ultimately, His Holiness himself, the Dalai Lama. Her exploration of self-realization continues today.

Ora lives with her husband, Jeff, and two sons, Jake and Benjamin in Los Angeles.

CPSIA information can be obtained
at www.ICGtesting.com
Printed in the USA
BVHW030206290319
543848BV00058B/858/P